# YOGA BODY
## ANATOMY

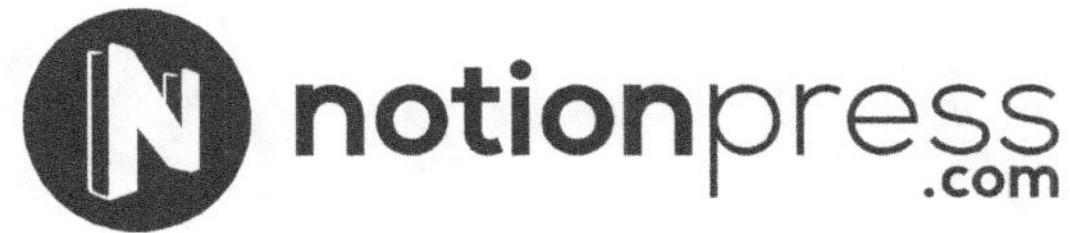

notionpress.com

# YOGA BODY ANATOMY

## INSIGHTS TO MUSCULAR MOVEMENTS

Dr. SHASHIREKHA C.K.

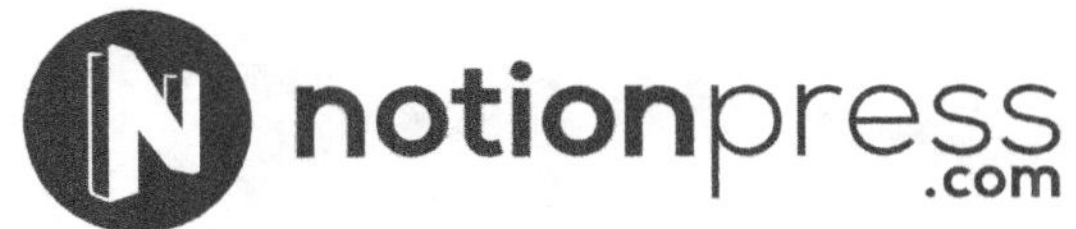

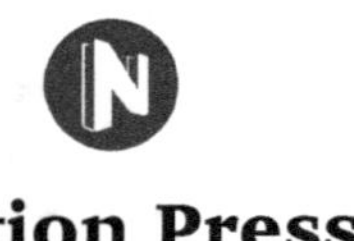

## Notion Press

Old No. 38, New No. 6
McNichols Road, Chetpet
Chennai - 600 031

First Published by Notion Press 2017
Copyright © Dr. Shashirekha C. K. 2017
All Rights Reserved.

ISBN  978-1-948146-49-4

*Dedicated to my parents, who guided me lovingly,
shared my life with joy and enthusiasm,
supported my academic and personal interests
and always thought the best of me.*

# CONTENTS


*Preface*                                                                                                                  *ix*

*Acknowledgement*                                                                                         *xiii*

*Introduction*                                                                                                  *xv*

**Chapter 1:** Connective Tissues                                                                1

**Chapter 2:** The Fundamentals of Yoga Practice: Breath, Bandha, Drishti and Vinyasa        63

**Chapter 3:** Asana Kinesiology                                                                 92

**Chapter 4:** Pranayama (Conscious Breathing)                                       102

**Chapter 5:** Asana Practice and the Importance of Maintaining Digestive Health        114

**Chapter 6:** Yoga Chikitsa—an Introduction to Yoga Therapy              128

**Chapter 7:** Meditation and Relaxation                                                 142

# PREFACE

It has been 9 years since I completed my post-graduation from the most prestigious Ayurveda institution in South India, the Government Ayurveda Medical College, Mysore, Karnataka, India. I had an avid interest in the origin and influence of this healing system and took every opportunity to delve into the original ancient texts for evidence of its philosophical and intellectual connections. For example, we know from archeological evidence that Ayurveda can be traced to the ancient cities of Mohenjo-Daro and Harappa in the region known as the Indus valley. At that time, a system of healing prevailed among the people known as Aryans in which sophisticated medicines of vegetable, animal and mineral origin were used. The Rigveda, the oldest known document from the Aryan civilization, contains abundant references to plants and herbal medicines. The concept of agni and soma, the seed concepts for lateral medical theories of digestion and reproduction, are likewise used in detail in this ancient metrical scripture. The Rigveda and two other early vedas (Yajurveda and Samaveda) are distinctly ritualistic and magical, full of references to sacrifice and deities. The deities were often personifications of natural forces, such as Sun, Wind and Earth. The later text of the vedic period, the Atharvaveda, provides a much more specific and detailed view of medicine as it existed in ancient India. The detailed description of the human body is an evidence of a highly developed knowledge of anatomy.

In addition, we find a great many disease conditions delineated, including hridroga (heart diseases), kushta (leprosy), rajayakshma (tuberculosis), ashmari (kidney stones) and unmada (insanity). There is also mention of many plants used in the treatment of specific diseases. Certainly, Ayurveda has its roots in this Atharvaveda era.

Gradually, with the dawning of scientific thought, these early vedic concepts of anatomy, physiology and pharmacology were greatly expanded and developed. Finally, during the first and second centuries AD, these ideas were organized and recorded as the famous encyclopedic compendiums of Charaka and Sushrutha. Even today, these books are regarded as the main textbooks of Indian medicine. It was during this period that Ayurvedic scholars began to incorporate ideas from schools of thought other than the Samkhya doctrine that was its main affiliation—one of these was the yoga school, the most celebrated and earliest texts of which is ascribed to Patanjali, a sage who lived during the end of second century AD. This school set forth the concept of the psychophysiological constitution of human beings, a system of controlling the mind and body through physical and behavioral disciplines, and methods of attaining one-pointed concentration. This latter goal could lead the aspirant to knowledge of the spirit untainted by matter.

Although it is commonly assumed that Patanjali was the founder of the yoga system, his own compendium, *Yoga Sutra*, states he was only the compiler and editor. The origin of the yoga system is more accurately ascribed to more ancient priest-physicians of the vedic era. The language of yoga has arisen from anatomical experimentations of various asanas on a laboratory called the human body by millions of sages over thousands of years. The system of yoga, although popularized in the West as a system of physical asanas, was originally considered medical in its purpose. The yoga system speaks about understanding diseases, its etiology, the course of the diseases and the methods to best eliminate it. This is in close agreement with the Ayurvedic approach to diseases. Clearly, Charaka (father of Indian medicine) was greatly influenced by the yoga school. Among the health-promoting measures common to yoga and Ayurveda are the use of mantras (chanting), diet, fasting, controlled breathing, relaxation, attending to natural urges in time and abstinence from excess and immoral behavior. Perhaps the most important link, however, is their common grounding in the text of the Samkhya philosophy. For example, there is a discussion in *Charaka Samhita* on the relationship between yoga and moksha (CS 2: 137–156). Moksha is defined by Charaka as the "complete annihilation of all material attachments"—moksha nivrittirnihsesha. Chakrapani, another noted ayurvedic commentator defines moksha as "absolute annihilation of the body"—atyantika sariradyucchedeh. Both these physicians identify yoga as the means of attaining this ultimate state of human liberation. Patanjali takes this idea further and provides the practical means, beginning with his second sutra: "Yoga chitta vritti nirodhah" (Yoga is the control of fluxes in the mind).

Today, there is a great need to clearly elucidate the therapeutic applications of yoga and its asanas. Although much is known, not much is written about the uses of asanas in the treatment of specific diseases. Among informed ayurvedic physicians interested in well-founded yoga research, the consensus is that 3 Indian institutions are conducting well-designed yoga research. Of the 3, the most respected is the Krishnamacharya Yoga Mandiram in Chennai. Other renowned institutions include the Kaivalyadhama Samithi Yogic Health Centre in Lonavia and the Sri Vivekananda Yoga Kendra in Bangalore. I personally opine that the limitations in these researches have a notable lack of correlation with modern medical understanding of diseases. Another limitation is that often the recommended asanas are beyond the ability of the individual in need, where help of some properties and preliminary exercises is needed to better accommodate the posture.

The message of yoga according to Patanjali is, "Prayatna saithilyaananta sampattibhyam" (YS 2:47), which means that the force and effort expended in doing asanas should be minimum. The postures are intended to be comfortable and steady (Sthiram sukham asanam, YS 2:46). The third limitation of yoga instructions is the emphasis on the achievement of a fixed, rigid form of each asana; this negates the individual constitutional differences of each practitioner and can even be injurious. Finally, the importance of breath as the key to one's yoga practice is often not emphasized enough.

So, in this book, I have sincerely attempted to address all these issues which certainly fulfill the need of a beginner of asana practice. I have taken into account the practical knowledge of enlivening all aspects of physiology. Take time to digest the words; practice the postures and breathing techniques as you proceed. This book will guide you with refreshing insight, born out of years of experience in treating diseases through a holistic approach and the challenge of self-discovery. With some perseverance and much letting-go, you will be amply rewarded.

May the next step on your journey in the path of yoga bring surprise and delight.

# ACKNOWLEDGEMENT

Most of what I learned about the meaning of yoga, its practice and the methods of yoga therapy I did during my graduation and post-graduation in Ayurvedic medicine.

Later, I started teaching these subjects along with yoga anatomy to aspiring teachers of yoga as part of the curriculum of their teacher training program. I am continually grateful to every student of mine for their trust and inspiration. I also want to acknowledge all of them for their patience with me as I honed my teaching skills.

It has been a privilege to put down my views on Yoga Anatomy. Teaching anatomy to the students of yoga and consulting them on various injuries during yoga practice brought to the fore many significant questions. All those questions, comments or even looks of utter confusion offered an opportunity for me to refine my teaching skills year after year. I thank all those students and appreciate their valuable feedback and interactions.

I am deeply grateful to my beloved husband, Dr Girish D, who motivated me to pen this book. Writing such an exhaustive book has taken a lot of time and concentration. I wrote it as our son, Abhin G, grew through his ninth year. All his responsibilities were taken care of by my loving mother, Smt Parvathamma K. It was only through their loving support that I was able to complete this project.

I would also like to convey my loving thanks to my younger brother, Prithviraj CK, who has inspired me with his strong dedication towards achievements.

My special thanks to Mr Harish Bheemaiah, owner of The Mysore Mandala Yogashala and Spiritual Centre, Mysore for giving me the initial opportunity to teach these subjects in his yogashala. Many other yogashalas also warmly welcomed me to be a part of their teacher training programs and teach yoga anatomy to their students. All of them have helped to get this book into your hands as well.

I am grateful to Dr Mudduraj, Associate Professor, JSS Medical college, Mysore., for believing in my work and sparing his valuable time to read my script. I thank him for his valuable suggestions and corrections and for generously sharing his medical and yoga knowledge.

There are many people who have been a part of the realization of this book, like my publisher, who is extremely patient and put up with me going way over the deadline. To everyone who has played a part in making this book possible, thank you…

# INTRODUCTION

*Yogena Chittasya padena vacham*
*Malam shareerasya cha vaidyakena*
*Yopakarotam pravaram muneenam*
*Patanjalim pranjalim ranatosmi*
*Om shanti shanti shanthihi*

As yoga teachers, it is very helpful to use simple words to explain movements. But as practitioners, we should comprehend very deeply the intricacies and complexities of movement.

If we understand what is happening in the poses, we can describe the actions required to perform the poses without using contradictory language.

Remember, Patanjali was the father of 3 fields: Yoga, Ayurveda and Grammar. Learning to communicate with clarity and consistency is one of the ways in which we can continue the tradition of yoga that has been passed on for centuries.

## History of Yoga

Yoga is a great Indian form of healing at the physical, mental, emotional and spiritual levels.

### Historical Background of Yoga

- Veda (c 1500–c 500 BCE), sacred scripture as "revealed wisdom," in the form of poems or hymns based on mystical visions, ecstasies and insights.
- *The Bhagavad Gita* (200 BCE–100 CE, "Song of Lord" 2500 years ago) is embedded in one of the Hindu epics, *The Mahabharata*. Its mystical author, Vyasa, weaved spiritual teaching into the account of events leading up to the 18-day war itself and its aftermath.
- Upanishads (100 BCE–300 CE, Seat of Wise, 2000 years ago).
- *Yoga Sutra* (400 CE, Philosophy, 1800 years ago by Patanjali), classic form of yoga, systematic control of thoughts.
- Shankaracharya (1000 years ago), founder of 10 branches of ashrams in India: Sivananda/Yogananda/Siddha Yoga—4 paths of yoga/classic Hatha Yoga/Kriya Yoga/Integral Yoga/Sadhana Yoga.

- *Yoga Pradipika* (fourteenth century by Svatamarama).
- Modern yoga era began: Krishnamacharaya (100 years ago, modern yogi), Pattabhi Jois/BNS Iyengar/BKS Iyengar/Desikachar—Iyengar Yoga/Ashtanga Yoga/Vini Yoga—Anasura Yoga/Yin Yoga/Jivamukti Yoga/Power Yoga/Sadhana Yoga.

Since ancient times, the asanas have been defined in terms of relatively precise forms; by mastering these forms, an individual demonstrates his or her mastery of certain basic principles of movement. Yet, it was also generally understood that the practical application of these principles must be based on each individual's actual condition. An individual's way of doing each posture was therefore worked out between teacher and student. In this sense, the transformational value of a posture was always seen in relation to its function, not to its form.

Unfortunately, chief among the popular misconceptions about yoga (including among many practitioners and even yoga teachers) is the idea that the value of each posture lies in achieving its precise, fixed form. Thus, emphasis has too often been placed on superficial details of positioning and the development of the body in the direction of preconceived, external standards of perfection. The forms have been crystalized into rigid, static postures in which the living quality of the asana is lost. To correct this, we must engage in an understanding of functional anatomy-kinesiology involved in each posture.

To deepen your mind's interface with your body's anatomy, you can begin to apply the study of anatomy to understanding how muscles move joints and create function. This is the study of kinesiology. This is not the same as applied kinesiology (a chiropractic reflex treatment method). In kinesiology, we learn how specific muscles and joints react during movement. We can learn which muscles contract, which ones stretch and move too far or not far enough. It is ideal to be able to move each joint both independently and in combination with other motions.

Through this study, you can predict which yoga poses will be difficult. If you've had an injury or postural abnormality and know the structures involved and how they normally move, by the application of kinesiology, you can predetermine exercises that will need remedial work before you attempt more challenging and complex motions.

Since 1910, scientists of physical medicine have studied the normal range of motion. Acceptable standards for the direction of movement and mobility of each joint have been established in the professions of physical medicine, physical therapy and orthopedics. They differ slightly in terms of the amount of flexibility considered normal for each joint. Joints move through a specific range of motion, as delineated by studies of physical medicine and orthopedics. Motions within this optimal range maintain the natural flow of synovial fluid for lubrication of the joints, as well as normal strength and flexibility of the antagonistic muscles on opposite sides of the joint. When this range is exceeded, by overstretching, poor posture, injury or skeletal deformity, the joint becomes hyperextended, less stable and potentially more vulnerable to injury. Conversely, when the range of a joint has been diminished, the resulting rigidity in the joint and postural muscles supporting it places more stress on neighboring joints and muscles. Every practitioner should be aware of these sequential changes which happen to the body on the yoga mat.

So, the aim of this book is to be as practical as possible in terms of understanding the anatomical perspective of yoga asanas. As you read, allow your understanding of what anatomy means to expand. Explore your body as an integrated whole. As you practice, experience asanas not as individual postures but as elements related to one another in the context of a greater whole. This book will encourage you to explore your understanding of anatomy via the personal laboratory that is your body. As a result, you will become a more mindful practitioner and a better teacher. Now, let's begin the journey to explore the world of yoga anatomy.

## Anatomy, Kinesiology and Yoga

### Definition of Anatomy

Anatomy is a branch of science concerned with the bodily structure of humans, animals and other living organisms.

### Definition of Kinesiology

Kinesiology is the science of human movement.

### Relevance of Anatomy and Kinesiology to Yoga Teachers

Practitioners and teachers must have

- Precision in practice.
- Comprehension of cause and effect in practice.
- Clarity in verbal instruction.
- Avoidance of excessive demonstration in class.
- Comprehension of individual differences.

Yoga is a power that builds strength and confidence, improves the body's flexibility and balance and imparts spiritual peace and contentment to the mind. Beyond its attributes as preventive medicine, yoga helps to heal, aids in recovery from all minor to major illness and to cope with chronic problems like arthritis, multiple sclerosis and infection with HIV.

Yoga awakens something deep inside us—the true self. To delve deeply inside ourselves, we must journey within our physical bodies. Once there, we will not only understand our anatomy but also directly experience the reality that gives rise to the core concepts of yoga. The reason for this mutually illuminating relationship between yoga and anatomy is simple; the deepest principles of yoga are based on a subtle and profound appreciation of how the human system is constructed.

The subject of yoga is the self, and the self is an attribute of a physical body. The context that yoga directs for the study of anatomy is rooted in the exploration of how our life force expresses itself through the movements of the body, breath and mind.

The language of yoga has arisen from anatomical experimentations of various asanas on the laboratory called human body by millions of sages over thousands of years. The study of anatomy offers a solid grounding in the principles of the physical practice of (asanas) all systems of yoga. As yoga practice emphasizes the relationship of breath and the spine, we pay special attention to those systems. By viewing all other body structures in light of their relationship to the breath and spine, yoga becomes an integrating principle for the study of anatomy.

We also deal with the yogic perspective of dynamic inter-relationship between all body systems. The ancient yogis held the view that we have 3 bodies: physical, astral and causal. From this perspective, yoga anatomy is the study of the subtle currents of energy that move through the layers or sheaths of those 3 bodies.

Let's take up these things more practically. Consider yourself sitting in a class and listening to a lecture. You have a mind and body that are currently inhaling and exhaling in a gravitational field. Therefore, you can benefit immensely from a process that enables you to think more clearly, breath more effortlessly and move more efficiently. This is, in fact, our starting point and definition of yoga practice anatomically: the integration of mind, breath and body.

## Basic Premises to Be Kept in Mind

1. Focus your attention.
2. Be aware of your breath.
3. Build concentration.
4. Move into and out of posture.
5. Honor the suggestion of pain.
6. Cultivate regularity, enthusiasm and caution.
7. Take personal responsibility.
8. Cultivate patience.

# The 5 Points of Yoga

Yoga is a life of self-discipline based on the tenets of "simple living and high thinking." The body is a temple or vehicle for the soul, and has specific requirements that must be fulfilled for it to function smoothly. These requirements may be seen metaphorically in relationship to an automobile. A car requires 5 major elements: a lubricating system, a battery, a cooling system, fuel and a responsible driver behind the wheel.

## 1. Proper Exercise

Asana practice acts as a lubricating routine to the joints, muscles, ligaments, tendons and other parts of the body by increasing circulation and flexibility. Yoga considers the body a vehicle for the soul in its journey towards perfection; asanas are designed not only to develop the body, but also to broaden mental faculties and spiritual capacities. Your body is as young as your flexibility. Asanas also work on the internal machinery of the body: the glands, organs and muscular system. By practicing yoga asanas not merely as physical exercise but as an exercise of awareness of the muscles being used, of breathing and of relaxation, the mind is detached from the senses little by little.

## 2. Proper Breathing (PrāNāYāMa)

This aids the body in connecting to its battery: the solar plexus, where tremendous potential energy is stored. When tapped through specific yoga breathing techniques (**pranāyāma**), the energy is released for physical and mental rejuvenation. Control of the prana, or subtle energy, leads to control of the mind. The grossest manifestation of prana in the human body is the motion of the lungs. All diseases of the body can be destroyed at the root by controlling and regulating the prana. This is the secret knowledge of healing. The person who has abundant pranic energy radiates vitality and strength.

## 3. Proper Relaxation (SavāSana)

This cools down the system like the radiator of a car. When the body and mind are continually overworked, their efficiency diminishes. Relaxation is nature's way of recharging the body. Relaxation includes 3 parts: physical, mental and spiritual. Physical relaxation refers to relaxing the bodily system by using autosuggestion. One mental relaxation technique is breathing slowly and rhythmically for a few minutes when experiencing mental tension. One may experience a kind of floating sensation when mentally relaxed. Spiritual relaxation is not to identify the self with mind and body because there will be worries, sorrows, anxieties, fear and anger; a yogi identifies him/herself with the all-pervading, all-powerful, all-peaceful, and joyful self, or pure consciousness, within.

## 4. Proper Diet (Vegetarian)

This provides correct fuel for the body. Optimum utilization of food, air, water and sunlight is essential. There is a cycle in nature known as the "food cycle" or "food chain." The sun is the source of energy for all life on our planet; it is at the top of the food chain. The food at the top of the chain has the greatest life-promoting properties. All natural food has different properties of essential nutrients. Animal flesh is considered a secondary source of nutrition. A health motto is "eat to live, not live to eat."

## 5. Positive Thinking and Meditation (Vedanta and DhyāNa)

These put you in control. With positive thinking and meditation, the intellect is purified. The lower nature, the desires of the mind, is brought under conscious control through steadiness and concentration.

As practitioners, it is important that we do not get stuck in asana. There is a lifetime of work to do in fully understanding and experiencing these postures and studying anatomy can add to this natural emphasis on the physical. In summary, encourage yourself to explore the understanding of anatomy via the personal laboratory that is your own body. As a result, you will become a more mindful practitioner and a better teacher.

# Chapter 1

# CONNECTIVE TISSUES

Connective tissue is the basis of functional anatomy. Let's begin our exploration of anatomy with the tissues that exemplify the interconnected nature of all our body parts—connective tissues.

First, let us consider the anatomical structures that make movement possible. A fundamental type of tissue is called connective tissue. This serves to connect, support and bind body structures together. Examples include

- Cartilage
- Bone
- Muscles
- Ligaments
- Tendons
- Fascia
- Fat

Connective tissues are comprised of 2 proteins, collagen and elastin. Collagen is known for its strength and elastin, as you may have guessed from its name, for its elasticity; it's the more pliable and resilient stuff. Put them together in varying proportions and densities and you will get the amazing array of connective tissues we find throughout the body.

All connective tissues, except cartilage, have many blood and lymph vessels and nerves. A joint is the meeting of the ends of 2 bones. There are approximately 206 bones that meet at 180 joints. I say approximately, as anomalies are not uncommon in the human body; some people are blessed with additional bones, muscles, and/or joints. The ends of bones that meet at a joint are surrounded by a capsule. The terminal ends of the bones are covered with hyaline cartilage, which lubricates and protects the smooth surfaces for fluid articulation. This area also contains various sensory elements. The sensors give proprioceptive awareness to our brain via fine nerve fibers, so that we are kept constantly informed about movements and the position of each joint. The joint has its own stability, provided by another type of connective tissue called ligament. Ligaments are fibrous bands that allow certain motions and prevent others. They will be lax in the direction of motions they create and reach the limit of their mobility to restrict motions that would otherwise injure the joint or surrounding muscle tissue. Ligaments can be tightened by injury or repeated muscular contractions, as in developing muscular stamina. They can also be stretched, though usually only with effort applied consistently. Some physical medicine specialists object to yoga students holding stretches too long, thus creating stretch, not in the muscles, but in ligaments. They fear this training may be a source of additional patients and potential surgery.

Ligaments can also be torn by forced motions or accidents that go beyond normal joint mobility. "The muscles are protected from injury by two kinds of nerve cells," Evjenth writes, "muscle spindles and tendon spindles." Muscle spindles prevent muscle cells from stretching too much when an unexpected movement occurs. They do this by making the muscle contract. This happens automatically and protects the muscle from overstretching. Slow, intentional stretching is not prevented by the muscle spindles. Tendon spindles tell the brain, via nerve fibers, how tense the muscle is. If the tension gets too high, the tendon spindles send signals to stop the muscle from contracting. These signals make the muscle relax. About 30 percent of our nervous system enervates these structures, which are responsible for our underlying learned messages regarding our posture. Because these neurons are operating at a subconscious level and cannot be accessed by the mind, it is only through the breath that these structures will release and "reset" the concerned muscle to a happier state.

Here, I would like to mention an excellent point on the importance of breath awareness in learning to relax muscle tissue, heightening the awareness of the moment and maintaining the ideal of where one wants to go in yoga practice. It is important to distinguish between yoga and stretching. While stretching is a feeling sensation, classical yoga is not concerned with these sensations. The keywords in describing the physical sensations of yoga poses are steadiness, comfort and relaxation of effort, according to Patanjali, in *Yoga Sutra*. Nowhere does it say that yoga consists of stretching exercises. Many writers suggest engaging in conscious stretching, done to purposely lengthen a muscle by holding a stretching position with a high degree of tension for a sustained period of time. As a result, the muscles are in fact, injured. There is a resultant increase in muscle-resting length from the tearing of muscle fiber. This is not classical yoga. Many people are under the mistaken impression that yoga focuses on stretching muscle fiber.

## Muscle Tissue

There are 3 types of muscle tissue. The most common—comprising 99 percent of the body's muscle mass—make up approximately 430 skeletal muscles that attach the skeleton together and maintain postural integrity. These are also called voluntary muscles, as they are responsible for all types of controlled conscious motion. They are involved, however, in automatic reflex motions, such as running and walking. The next major group is smooth muscles, which make up many internal organs and blood vessels. The third group is the cardiac muscle, located only in the heart. Altogether, muscles make up about 60 percent of our body's mass. Crossing over each joint are one or more skeletal muscles. Motor nerves coming from the spinal cord activate skeletal muscles. An electrical impulse from the nerve endings spans the gap to the muscle surface via a chemical secretion of acetylcholine.

## *Types of Muscle Tissue*

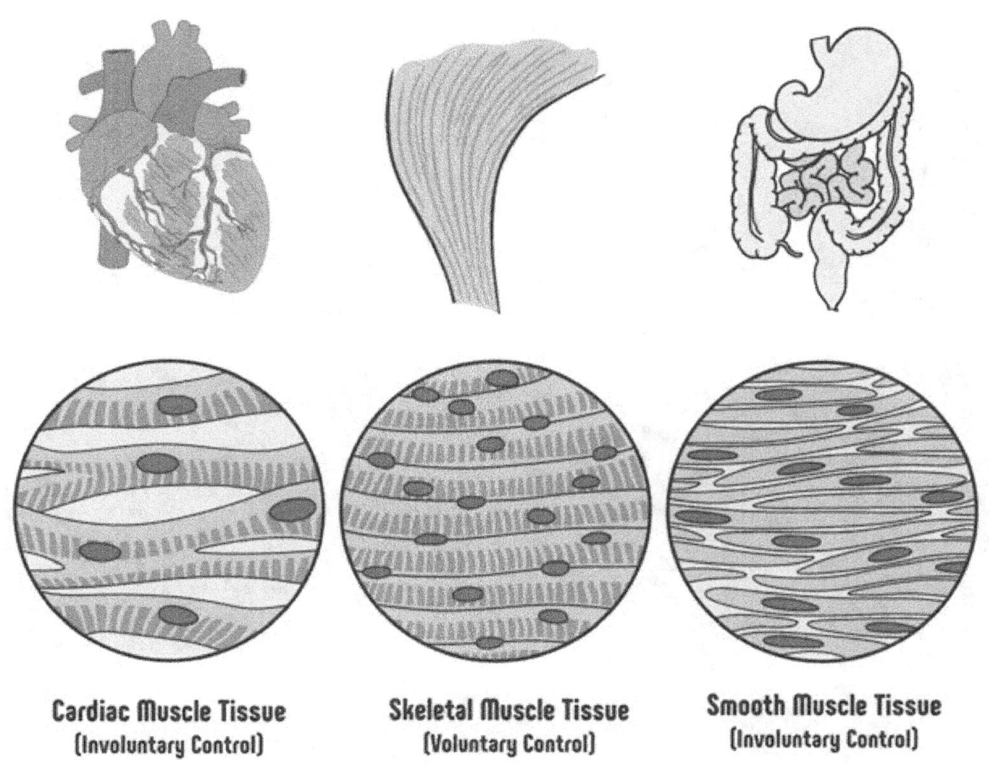



Diagram of types of muscle tissue

The muscle stays contracted until an enzyme that neutralizes acetylcholine is produced to create relaxation. Thus, muscles have only 2 properties—they contract, which strengthens them, or they relax. ndividual muscles can act only to shorten, and not to lengthen, the distance between two attachment points—they can pull but not push. For movement in the opposite direction, another muscle must be activated.

Skeletal muscles are made up of 2 types of fibers—dark or slow-twitch fibers and white or fast-twitch fibers. Thomas Griner says that only slow-twitch muscle fibers can metabolize fatty acids and that this is desirable for several reasons. First, fat metabolism is aerobic, burns cleanly and doesn't make lactic acid. It can also draw directly on stored body fat and help reduce it. The fast-twitch muscle fiber can only metabolize glucose. So, during heavy exercise, this process will be aerobic, but most of it will produce lactic acid and actually be anaerobic. The more vigorous your exercise program, the more you are engage fast-twitch fibers, while leaving the slow-twitch ones behind. This means you burn less fat and produce more lactic acid. Slow movement is of greater benefit since it uses both the fast- and slow-twitch fibers, thereby activating all muscles.

Slow steady-paced yoga practice, based on the Patanjali tradition, is an efficient form of exercise for burning fat and reducing lactic acid. Patanjali provides guidelines that, in effect, minimize the effort involved during the practice of asana. Scientific research has also discovered that this type of stretching, characterized by low force yet long duration, produces a plastic or permanent deformation in the muscle tissue. The opposite type of stretching, high force and short duration, was shown by the same researchers to produce elastic or recoverable deformation in muscle tissue.

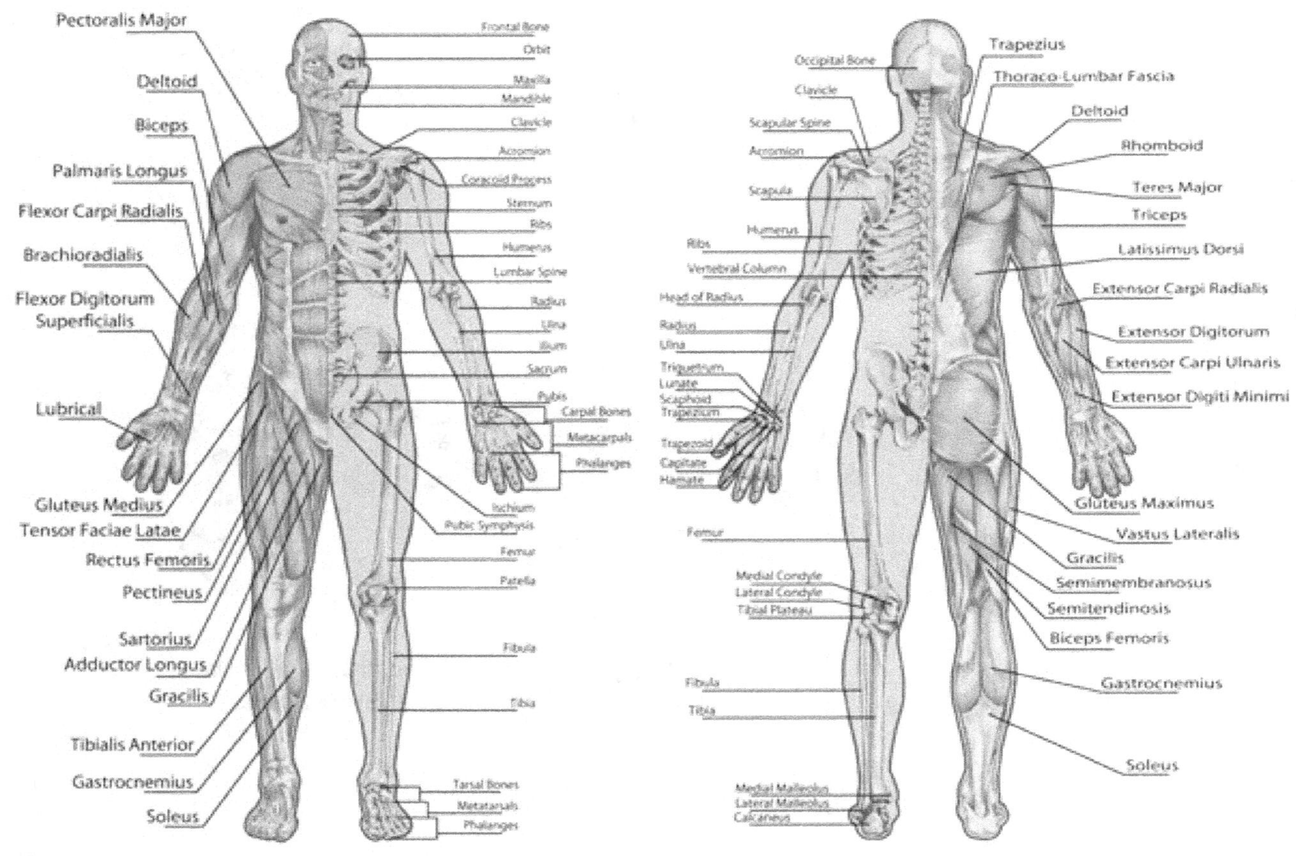

Diagram of the human musculoskeletal system

From the diagram above, you can make out the skeletal muscles attached to the bones. Skeletal muscles have at least 2 attachments. The attachment at either end of the muscle is called tendon. One end is connected to a more freely mobile limb called the insertion and the other to a less-moveable attachment called the origin. When a muscle contracts, it exerts a pull on both ends toward the middle of the belly of the muscle, which usually moves the insertion toward the origin. In the case of the biceps brachii, its origin is on the shoulder and insertion on the upper forearm. When it contracts, it pulls the forearm toward the shoulder, as in the action of picking up an object. This is the natural movement of the insertion moving toward the origin. It can also contract, by pulling the body toward the forearm, as in the pull-up or chin-up exercise motion. In this case, the origin is moving toward the insertion. Muscles have two basic ways of working:

1. Concentrically, when the muscle fibers contract or shorten so that the origin and insertion come closer to each other.

2. Eccentrically, when the muscle fibers lengthen so that the origin and insertion move away from each other. When a muscle contracts without changing its length, we call it isometric contraction.

Many muscles work in pairs. The muscle that contracts in the most direct line of a specific motion is called the agonist or the primary mover. Other muscles helping in the motion are called secondary movers. A muscle that relaxes to allow motion (this may be felt as a passive stretch) is called the antagonist. For instance, when the biceps brachii contracts, it bends/flexes the elbow. This can only happen if the antagonist muscle, the triceps brachii, relaxes/stretches. Conversely, to straighten/extend the elbow, the triceps brachii will contract, if the biceps brachii relaxes. Sometimes, the work of contraction is more than the muscle is accustomed to. Then, there will be a residual contraction. In the example above, if the biceps brachii is overworked, once relaxed, the elbow will remain partially flexed. Afterwards, you may find yourself complaining of stiffness in the biceps. This will commonly occur when a muscle has been used extensively. For instance, when you curl weight from a straight arm position, bringing it toward the shoulder, you contract the biceps strongly. After overexertion in building the muscle, the arm will hang at the side with a perpetual bend/flexion of the elbow joint. This is often the case with weightlifters who do not balance the full range of toning the triceps brachii with toning the biceps brachii. The residual contraction of the biceps has not been balanced relative to its antagonist muscle, the triceps. For the complete range of motion to occur, the triceps brachii must fully relax so that the biceps brachii can fully contract.

This is what we are seeking in yoga-based movements—a mobility that is within acceptable medical standards for joint health and is also smooth, steady and comfortable, to produce a heightened sensitivity. To understand the principle of antagonistic motion is to understand balance and symmetry. When any muscle is fully contracted, its antagonist muscle or muscles will necessarily be fully relaxed and stretched to their end points. This principle creates full range of motion. Whenever there is lack of mobility, there is necessarily an imbalance in antagonist muscles. The contracting muscle is weak and its antagonist is too tight. By getting to know the antagonist muscles, a student can learn to balance flexibility with strength.

During exercise, muscles must perform 2 main tasks:

1.  "burn" available fuel for energy and
2.  contract in response to a rush of electrical signals from the brain.

## Muscle Fuel during Exercise

Muscle can burn multiple fuels during exercise, including glucose (from carbohydrates), fatty acids (from fat) and amino acids (from protein). The type of fuel burned for energy depends on the intensity and duration of the exercise being performed.

In the same way that a car stores fuel in a fuel tank, muscles have evolved the ability to store glucose, fatty acids and amino acids on-board. All 3 fuels are burned for energy in the mitochondria, organelles within muscle cells that function much like a car engine.

### Glucose Is Stored as Glycogen

Glucose is stored within each muscle cell as glycogen. Glycogen is a quick-burning fuel used during high-intensity exercise.

## Fatty Acids Are Stored as Triglyceride

Fatty acids are stored within muscle cells as triglycerides. Triglycerides provide a secondary fuel source for low-intensity exercise.

## Amino Acids Are Stored as Muscle Protein

Finally, amino acids are stored within the muscle tissue as muscle protein itself. Unlike glucose and fatty acids, there is no storage tank for amino acids in the muscle tissue. The muscle itself is the amino acid storage tank.

Here's another way to visualize the storage tanks in muscle tissue:

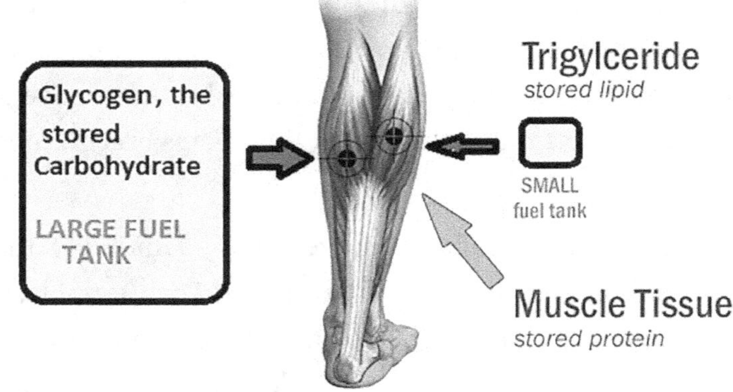


## The Choice of Fuel Depends on Exercise Intensity

As you can see in the graph below, as the intensity of exercise increases, the dependence on carbohydrate goes up and the dependence on fatty acids goes down. This means your muscles will use your glucose storage tank to fuel your workout so you can eat more carbs!

At low intensities, fatty acids are the main fuel source and only small amounts of glycogen are broken down. As the intensity of exercise increases, larger amounts of glycogen are broken down and burned for energy, making glucose the predominant fuel source.

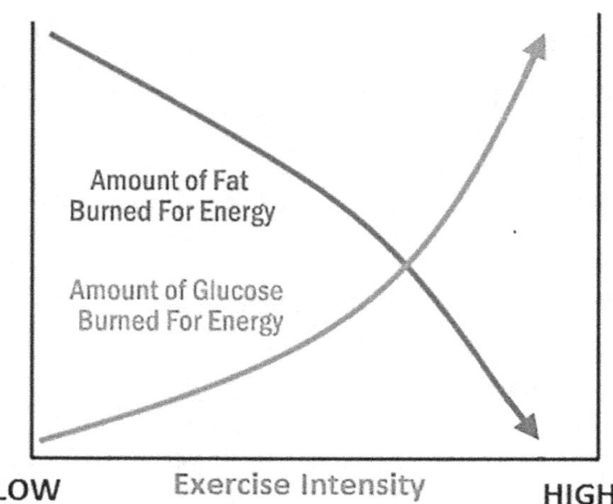


[6]

Amino acids from protein are the lowest priority fuel; given amino acids are the infrastructure of the muscle tissue itself. To preserve muscle mass, glucose and fatty acids will be burnt first, before resorting to amino acids.

## Muscle Micro Trauma

Although amino acids from muscle protein are the last choice for fuel during exercise, microscopic tears result from repeated muscle contractions, called micro trauma. These microscopic tears are one of the signals that the muscle needs repair during rest.

Think of micro trauma as the repeated wear and tear that your car experiences from driving long distances. In the same way that you replace damaged engine parts with newer and more efficient technology, micro trauma requires repair work immediately following exercise.

Recovery is a vital, often overlooked aspect of your workout regimen. It's very important to let your muscles rest and to replace your "fuel" with the right foods.

Let's get to know the different ways in which your muscles contract to power up your asana practice.

There's a reason your yoga teachers say things like, "Eccentrically contract your triceps to slowly lower into Chaturanga," instead of just, "Contract your triceps." It's because there are 3 different ways a muscle can contract and how you utilize these actions can affect strength and safety in a pose. So, what is really going on inside the muscle tissue when we flex and why does it matter?

## Three Types of Muscle Contractions

To get a feel for the mechanics in question, bend your elbow. The biceps on the front of your arm contracts to lift your forearm, creating a shortening of muscle fibers or concentric contraction. If you keep your elbow bent, your biceps stay contracted to resist gravity in a static (non-moving) or isometric contraction. Such contractions probably feel familiar—they're what you'd do if you wanted to "make a muscle."

Now, slowly lower your forearm. The triceps muscle on the back of your arm, which is responsible for straightening your elbow, is working now. However, because gravity pulls your forearm down, your triceps doesn't need to do anything. Rather, your biceps continue to contract as it lengthens, resisting gravity. If it didn't, your forearm would simply fall. Such lengthening, or eccentric contractions, are critical to controlling many movements, from folding forward into Uttanasana (Standing Forward Bend) to jumping back to Chaturanga Dandasana (Four-Limbed Staff Pose) to moving into an arm balance like Parshwabakasana (Side Crane Pose).

Use all 3 muscle contractions in your yoga practice.

Targeting concentric, isometric and eccentric contractions in your asana practice will work your muscles through their full range of motion, helping you to develop balanced strength and lessening your risk of injury. To understand these contractions, you need to know what happens in your muscles when they're working. Muscle cells, or fibers, contain many smaller strands called myofibrils, each of which in turn comprises a series of contractile units called sarcomeres. Within the sarcomere,

2 types of protein filaments—thick filaments called myosin and thin filaments called actin—overlap like interlaced fingers.

When a muscle like the biceps contracts concentrically, a signal from the central nervous system prompts the thick myosin filaments to hold on to nearby thinner actin filaments, forming linkages called cross-bridges. If the pull is strong enough to overcome opposing resistance (usually from the force of gravity), the actin strands slide between the myosin filaments and the muscle shortens—in this case, pulling up your forearm.

A similar thing happens during an isometric contraction, except the force generated by the myosin cross-bridges exactly matches the opposing resistance, so there is no movement and your arm stays fixed.

If the resistance is greater than the force the muscle generates, such as what happens to the biceps when lowering from a pull-up, the biceps muscle will be stretched, producing an eccentric contraction that allows your arm to lengthen with control. Scientists don't yet fully understand this process, but it seems that during an eccentric contraction, some myosin cross-bridges continue to latch onto actin filaments, while others are pulled apart.

Perhaps, surprisingly, muscles generate more force eccentrically than concentrically, meaning you can lower a heavier weight than you can lift. You can use this principle to build strength by focusing on lowering movements. For instance, controlling the descent from Plank Pose to Chaturanga will eccentrically contract and strengthen your triceps, while pushing back up to Plank is a concentric contraction of your triceps.

Because eccentric contractions produce more force than concentric ones, they also put more stress on muscles. If you're not used to it, eccentric exercise can damage muscle proteins, triggering delayed-onset muscle soreness or DOMS—usually at its worst 1–2 days after a tough workout. While DOMS may be annoying, it is rarely serious. Your muscles adapt by becoming stronger after a bout of DOMS, so that the next time you do the same routine, you are less likely to be sore.

Another caveat about eccentric exercise is that it may also stress tendons, the connective tissue that binds muscles to bones. Repeatedly overloading your tendons in this way without allowing for recovery increases your risk of tendon damage, or tendinopathy, a painful condition that can interfere with your practice. Due to their slow metabolic rate, tendons recover gradually; once tendinopathy develops, it can take months for full recovery.

That doesn't mean you should avoid eccentric exercise. In fact, strengthening your muscles eccentrically will help build stronger, more resilient muscles and tendons that are less likely to get injured in the future—as long as you allow them to adapt slowly. In fact, physical therapists frequently use eccentric exercises to rehab injured tendons.

Exploring the entry into side crane pose will help us understand how to use eccentric contractions wisely in your yoga practice.

### *How to Use Eccentric Contractions in Parshwa Bakasana (Side Crane Pose)?*

The transition into an arm balance like the Side Crane Pose can be scary. There is a very real risk of falling on your head, given that one arm is supporting most of your weight. Eccentrically engaging your triceps will allow you to come into the pose safely and with control, avoiding a painful face plant.

Squat with your feet and knees together, then twist your upper body to the right, bringing your left upper arm against the outside of your right knee. Place your hands on the floor alongside your right thigh, shoulder-width apart. As you shift your weight forward onto your hands, lift your feet. Imagine that you are pressing the floor away with your hands. This will keep your triceps eccentrically engaged as your elbows bend, controlling how far your head lowers toward the floor.

When you find your balance, your triceps muscles will work isometrically to keep you there. However, at the sweet spot where your upper and lower body exactly counterweight each other—like the 2 arms of a scale—your triceps won't need to do much. If you sense yourself falling forward, lightly press the floor away with your fingers, concentrically contracting your triceps to return to the balance point. Eventually, as you get stronger, you can work toward straightening your elbows by further concentrically engaging your triceps.

## Questions and Answers

Here, I have featured some common questions and answers about muscles and bone tissue generally asked by students.

**1. My muscles shake during certain poses. Is it safe to keep holding them?**

Answer: Yes, to an extent. Shaking or quivering muscles during difficult yoga poses are a physiological and neurological response to working hard, and signal muscular fatigue, which is usually a good thing! Don't shy away from a pose when your muscles start to contract and relax, but do be mindful; if your alignment degrades, it can increase the risk of injury. To gauge the difference, listen to your teacher's cues and focus on your breath. If you can't inhale and exhale smoothly or if you start to hold or restrict your breath, your body is saying it has had enough and your alignment could be compromised; it's time to move out of the pose.

Another reason muscles may shake during difficult poses is dehydration, which throws off the balance of electrolytes like sodium and potassium that carry electrical impulses and allow your muscles to contract. The result: your muscles can't fire correctly and they quiver. If you're doing strenuous practice for more than 60 minutes, prevent quaking muscles by adding electrolytes: sip about 20 ounces of an electrolyte-containing beverage 2 to 3 hours before practice.

**2. What should I do if I experience pain during yoga class?**

Answer: If you feel discomfort beyond typical muscle fatigue, such as sudden and sharp pain, that may indicate a serious injury. Gently get out of the pose and tell your teacher. Often, pain in a pose can be alleviated with a simple modification or a supportive prop like a block. If the pain persists or worsens or it's too severe to continue, stop your practice and seek the advice of a medical professional.

### 3. My lower back often hurts after big backbends. How can I protect myself?

Answer: When a specific body region consistently experiences pain in asana practice, it's possible that the area is being asked to do too much range of motion or too much work or both. During backbends, you may be pushing yourself to move too far in space, as opposed to making all the little articulations available in your spine. Experiment with letting your lower spine be the last part of your spine to move into a big backbend, which may help redistribute the stresses of the movement. Use your breath to explore both the depth and width of your rib cage. This will help you find the stiffer places in your thoracic region that may not be fully participating in the extension. Also, although inhaling lifts and opens the rib cage, it puts the thoracic spine into flexion (forward bending). For many people, exhaling into a deep backbend provides significant relief from lower-spine strain.

If one of your "big backbends" is the Wheel Pose, pay attention to your legs. When entering the Wheel Pose from a supine position, focus on pulling with the legs rather than pushing. If your legs push (weight toward your toes rather than your heels), the Wheel Pose will not only overtax your arms, but will also compress the lower spine; pulling does the opposite.

All said, everyone experiences postures differently, and chronic pain should be taken seriously. So, consult a health care practitioner if discomfort persists.

### 4. I have very tight hips, and I often feel pressure on my knee when entering the Pigeon Pose. How can I avoid this?

Answer: Any painful sensation in the knee joint should be taken very seriously. I'll assume you're free from any knee conditions and injuries, that the pressure is in the front of the knee and that you're practicing the most common version of the pose, in which the back leg is extended behind you, the spine is upright, and the fingertips press into the floor. This is actually a modification of Eka Pada Rajakapotanasana (Pigeon Pose).

Before attempting this variation, it's wise to warm up the hip rotators and associated muscles. Start your practice with standing poses like Vrkshasana (Tree Pose) and Virabhadrasana (Warrior Pose) I, II and III. Then, practice Baddha Konasana (Bound Angle Pose) to externally open the hip joint. Move into Ardha Matsyendrasana (Half Lord of the Fishes Pose) and increase the hip rotator stretch by drawing the top of the knee into your chest. Lastly, try Gomukhasana (Cow Face Pose), leaning forward to increase the action in the hips.

When you're ready to try the modified version of Eka Pada Rajakapotanasana, place a folded blanket under the hip of the front leg. Also, you will sometimes hear the instruction to pull the front heel away from the groin so the shin is parallel to the front of your mat; in your case, I recommend keeping the front heel close to the groin. Both of these actions will reduce the amount of rotation required of the hip, which should lessen the chance of pinching the tissues in your knee.

If you still don't find relief, I recommend that you discontinue this pose until you can find a qualified yoga teacher to help you adapt it to your body. In the meantime, there are many preparatory poses you can work on to open the hips.

**5. Are the popping, cracking joints you hear while practicing yoga problematic or not?**

Answer: Cracking and popping noises can be attributed to a few different phenomena. One explanation is that when a joint is pushed into or out of its normal position (which could be done during a yoga pose) gases, primarily nitrogen, are displaced and escape from the synovial fluid inside the joint, causing a popping sound.

Another reason for these sounds is a tendon moving across a joint or from arthritic changes that have already occurred in the joint. If this popping occurs naturally during yoga practice, or in daily life for that matter, there is no problem. If the popping is from a tendon moving across a joint or from arthritis, continue to pay attention to the area, and if the symptoms change or if there is pain associated with the popping or cracking noise, seek the counsel of a qualified health professional.

However, it is unadvisable to continually try to pop one's joints (that is, cracking the knuckles). This practice tends to create hypermobility and can lead to instability in the joint. This instability can cause the surrounding musculature to tighten up to support the joint and thus the urge to pop will arise again.

**6. I have tight hamstrings. How can I release them?**

Answer: You're not alone. Tight hamstrings are a very common issue, but you can do something about it. Stretching regularly actually does make them more flexible, and this sequence is all you need. As a bonus, it'll target the muscles in the lower back and hips as well. Complete the following sequence once with the right leg and then again with the left.

## Seated Straddle

Begin by sitting on the floor with the legs out wide. With straight legs and a straight back, slowly hinge at the hips, reaching out with the chest to prevent the spine from rounding. Rest your hands on your thighs or on the floor. Only fold as far as you can with straight legs and hold here for 5 breaths (about 30 seconds).

## Seated Straddle

Take this pose a little deeper by reaching your hands down the legs. Make sure to keep the legs straight and rest the hands on the thighs, knees, shins or if you can, reach for the big toes. With shoulders relaxed, breathe deeply for 5 breaths, using the ab muscles to pull the torso closer to the floor.

## 1-Legged Seated Straddle

While in the seated straddle position, walk the hands over to the right leg. Try to bring each shoulder on either side of the thigh. Rest the hands on the floor or on the leg. After 5 breaths, walk your hands over to the left leg for another 5 breaths.

## Butterfly

Bend the knees and bring the soles of the feet together. Rest your hands on the feet, or to deepen the stretch, bring the hands underneath the calves and use your upper body to pull the torso and head toward the floor. Enjoy this hip stretch for 5 breaths.

## Seated Forward Bend Relaxed

Extend the legs out in front of you. With the legs and back straight, hinge at the hips, walking the hands toward the feet, either sliding them down the legs or on the floor on either side of the legs. Actively draw the shoulders back and down, away from the ears. Enjoy this stretch for 5 breaths.

## Modified Heron Pose

Sit with the legs extended in front of you. Bend the right knee and hold onto the back of the right thigh, the calf or if you can, the right heel. With the left leg straight and the foot flexed, straighten the right leg as much as you can, reaching the chest toward the ceiling. Hold this pose for 5 breaths.

## Modified Side Heron Pose

From the Modified Heron Pose, take the right leg out to the side, holding the thigh, calf or heel. If it's too difficult with the right leg extended in the air, just bend the knee and rest the foot on the floor. Rest your left hand on the floor for support. Gaze to the left for the duration of 5 breaths.

## Modified Heron Spinal Twist

From the Modified Side Heron Pose, bring your left hand to the right outer ankle. Keep the right knee bent if you need to and work on straightening the leg. Rest your right hand on the floor behind you for support and to help encourage a deeper twist. Lift the chest high and hold for 5 deep breaths.

## Rock the Baby

From the Modified Heron Spinal Twist, rotate the torso back to the center. Bend the right knee and place the right heel in the crook of your left elbow and the right knee in the crook of the right elbow. Sitting tall, hug the lower leg as close as you can to the chest. Enjoy this hip opener for 5 breaths.

## Overstretched Hamstrings

**7. I practice Ashtanga yoga and have developed a very painful ache around my sit bone area. I've tried to bend my knees in forward bends, but this makes the pain worse. Now, even walking can set off the ache. Can you suggest anything?**

Answer: The area around the sit bone is where the hamstrings originate and insert into the head of the femur or thighbone. This nagging and all-too-common injury typically occurs when the belly of the muscle doesn't stretch sufficiently, forcing the origin—the point where muscle becomes tendon—to compensate by overstretching.

A rule of thumb in yoga practice is that when you go too far in one direction, the way to fix it is by doing the opposite movement. When a muscle or tendon stretches, it weakens, and when it overstretches to the point of injury, it becomes very weak. To strengthen the injured area, you need to contract it. Some asanas that strengthen the origin of the hamstrings are Purvottanasana (Intense Front-Body Stretch) and Salabhasana (Locust Pose).

Avoiding forward bends entirely makes it difficult to practice. So, try doing forward bends with the quadriceps firmly engaged and contracted to encourage the lengthening of the belly of the hamstrings. When the quadriceps contract, the knee joint extends and the knee is straight, which is why bending your knees will not be helpful. Bending your knees in forward bends makes it impossible for the quadriceps to fully engage and only shortens the belly of the muscle, putting more strain at the origin of the hamstrings.

One way of working with this injury in seated forward bends is to make an eccentric contraction of the hamstrings. Unlike a normal contraction, when a muscle shortens, in an eccentric contraction, a muscle lengthens as it contracts. An eccentric contraction requires great strength in a muscle. In this case, it will strengthen the injured area while maintaining flexibility.

Sit in Pashchimottanasana (Seated Forward Bend) with your feet pressed against a wall. Press against the floor with the back side of the injured leg while pressing into a wall with the foot of this leg. As you press the ball of the foot against the wall, contract the quadriceps, and as you press the heel against the wall, contract the hamstrings. On the inhalation press strongly with the back of the leg against the floor and with the foot against the wall. As you exhale, increase the forward bend slightly while maintaining the resistance.

To do standing poses, try cinching a belt tightly around the injured area for support and awareness. You can also help break up the scar tissue at the injured area by placing a small ball under the site and rolling on it. Create hamstring strength to prevent strain with yoga poses that develop the muscles and tendons. There's nothing like a good stretch to ease stiff, sore muscles, right? Except when it makes things worse, which can happen if that tender spot is signaling a muscle tear.

Surprisingly, hamstring tears and strains happen quite often to yoga practitioners because of repetitive overstretching, especially when combined with insufficient strength in the muscle to counterbalance flexibility. Overstretching can cause micro-trauma or small tears (versus a big trauma like a large tear from a fall) in muscle, ligament, tendon or other soft tissue of the musculoskeletal system. And once you're injured, ongoing stretching can prevent healing, setting the stage for chronic or recurrent inflammation and pain, and making the affected tissue vulnerable to further tearing.

If you study common practice sequences, you'll see that it's easy to overdo stretching. Many sequences contain a high percentage of hamstring stretches, including some standing poses, standing forward bends, seated forward bends and other back-of-the-leg stretches. On the other hand, hamstring-strengthening poses are typically practiced less often, so we're missing out on their ability to build endurance in the actual muscle fibers. Working the muscle also creates strength and toughness in the tendons that attach the muscle to the bone, making them less likely to strain and tear.

Let's take a closer look at the 3 hamstring muscles. Each originates (attaches) on the sitting bones of the pelvis and runs down the back of the thigh.

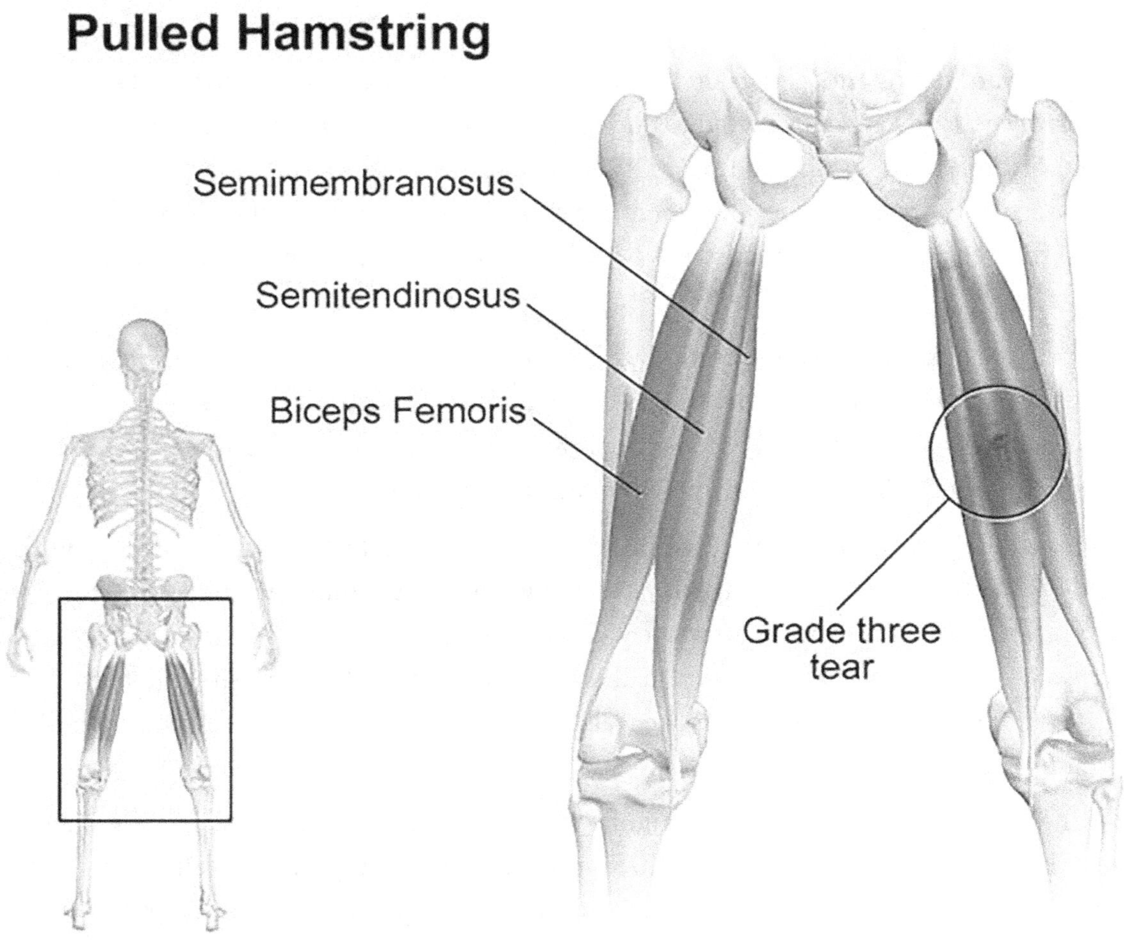


There are 2 hamstrings on the medial (inner) side of the back of the thigh and one on the lateral (outer) side; all 3 are attached by long tendons crossing the back of the knee to the lower leg. Usually, a bit of mid-muscle discomfort on the back of the thigh won't cause problems. However, pay attention if you feel discomfort or pain near the sitting bones as you stretch or if you find it painful to sit for extended periods, especially on a hard surface. If this is the case, stretching the hamstrings during your practice will leave them sorer afterward, due to renewed microscopic tearing and painful inflammation.

If you suspect you have strained or torn your hamstring through excessive stretching, it's time to change your practice to avoid constant re-injury and to facilitate healing. As is probably obvious by now, you have to stop stretching your hamstrings—this could be for just a few weeks or in more serious cases, a few months. Students often object, but unless you want a chronic or recurrent problem, you simply need to give the tissues time to heal. However, you don't have to halt yoga entirely; you could practice poses for upper-body strength or quadriceps flexibility. Once the tear has healed—that means a week or two with little or no pain—you can gradually resume stretching, but start gently, with only one pain-free stretch at a time.

Even while the hamstrings are healing, you can begin strengthening them about every other day (once a week isn't enough to build strength). Strengthening increases blood flow, and a good blood supply promotes healing and makes for healthier, more resilient tissue. However, pain is a sign that the tissues are still too inflamed and won't be able to bear the load without further irritation. In this case, you may need to wait a bit longer after you stop stretching to begin strengthening.

When you're ready, you can easily start traditional resistance training at home, with a light ankle weight of 2–3 pounds. Lie on your stomach with your legs straight out behind you on the floor. Bend your knee at a 90-degree angle, with your shin perpendicular to the floor and your thigh on the floor, then lower your foot back down. Complete 10 repetitions, smoothly and slowly, and gradually build to 3 sets of 10 reps.

To work on hamstring-strengthening yoga poses, focus on bent-leg standing poses like Virabhadrasana I and II (Warrior Pose I and II) and Utthita Parsvakonasana (Extended Side Angle Pose). Most yoga practitioners are aware that the quadriceps on the front of the thigh are working hard in these poses, but the hamstrings are working too, co-contracting with the quads of the bent knee to stabilize that hip and knee against the pull of gravity. Be sure to use a timer to help you gradually build your hold time—you could start with 15 seconds and build to 1 minute—as holding these poses builds quality isometric strength. Working a muscle isometrically, or contracting without changing the muscle's length, trains it to "hold" and stabilize, an important function for general posture and for any poses requiring you to hold your body weight for more than a few seconds against gravity.

You can also strengthen the hamstrings during hip extensions in such poses as Salabhasana (Locust Pose) as you lift the whole leg off the floor, and Setu Bandha Sarvangasana (Bridge Pose). These hip-extending poses put more load on the upper part of the hamstring, likely helping to increase strength and bulk in the strained area at the sitting bones.

As your injured hamstring heals—and be patient, as it may take several weeks—gradually rebuild your asana practice, so that you have a good balance of hamstring-strengthening and -stretching poses. Try doing some of the hamstring-strengthening poses in the first part of your practice, and then stretching them afterward when the muscles are warm and tired and ready to relax. Or, you can focus on the strengthening poses one day and work on deep stretching the next. Your goal for optimal health is to cultivate muscles that are strong and flexible and able to support your joints fully, while still allowing a full range of motion in a wonderful variety of poses.

Practice the Bridge Pose for stronger hamstrings: The Bridge Pose is a very effective hamstring-strengthening posture. The hamstrings work hard to lift the pelvis off the floor and help to build the arch of this beginning backbend. Practicing some bent-leg standing poses (remember those Warriors!) is a great way to warm up for Bridge. Then, lie on your back, with knees bent and feet flat and pulled in close to your hips. Make sure your feet are parallel: feet and knees turning out can contribute to knee and back pain. To get the best possible contraction from your hamstrings, start by lifting only your tailbone off the floor, while leaving your sacrum and lower back on the floor. Imagine your pelvis is being pulled up by a string attached to your pubic bones, creating a posterior pelvic tilt. (Lifting from your navel elicits almost no contraction by the hamstrings and leaves the tailbone to hang down, creating lower-back discomfort and anterior pelvic tilt—the opposite of what you want.) Once you've started the lift from the tailbone, continue to roll up sequentially, from the sacrum to the lumbar vertebrae to the mid-back, coming into full Bridge or one of the variations that follow.

Variations: If you have arthritis, disc injuries or other lower-back problems and want to avoid backbends, you can stop at the Half Bridge Pose, forming a straight line from shoulder to hip to knee. Without putting any backbend in your spine, your hamstrings will be working hard to hold up your pelvis and press the pubic bones toward the ceiling. Or, if your back is healthy, you can continue rolling up into full Bridge, opening your chest and eventually lifting up enough to place your palms on your back ribs, fingers pointing toward the spine. Continue using your legs to lift the pelvis, which not only strengthens the hamstrings but also helps take weight off your wrists. For additional hamstring focus, put a belt around the front of your ankles and hold the ends with your hands near your ankles. Once you're up in the pose, pull on the belt as you try to draw the tops of your shins toward your hips. Roll up and down 3–4 times, gradually building your hold to a full minute or more each time. Do this sequence a few times a week and you'll be well on your way to stronger, pain-free hamstrings.

A common problem we all face is maintaining the health of our muscle tissue. Since muscles comprise so much of our body, nearly three-fifths of our mass, their health has a direct effect on the nervous system and the circulatory system and impacts every function of the body, every organ and gland. When a muscle is in spasm, it adversely affects nerves and blood vessels and is a crucial, though little understood, factor in illness and disease. When excess lactic acid becomes trapped in a muscle, it will eventually develop an abnormal, sustained contraction known as hypertonic spasm. It is extremely important to realize that we all have muscles in spasm. Although spasm causes pain, most of us are not aware of it. This is because when muscles become spastic, the body releases its own painkillers called endorphins. Endorphins block the pain of muscle spasm from reaching your brain.

The spasms can be bad as they can cut off circulation and sensation in nearby nerves. The nerves become blocked and you don't feel any pain because the area is numb. Muscle spasm can create other physical problems, whether or not you feel the pain. You may develop bone, muscle and joint problems, as well as other problems ranging from allergies to blocked arteries. You may experience cramps or tics, or more violent muscle spasms.

There are 2 types of skeletal muscles: flat and round. Flat skeletal muscles and their tendons are arranged in sheets that attach to the bone in a line. The tension is distributed evenly in a plane when a flat muscle contracts. Flat muscles are not subject to insidious spasm because they cannot trap lactic acid. Examples of flat muscles are the latissimus dorsi of the middle and lower back and the gluteus maximus of the buttocks. Round muscles and their tendons attach to bone between 2 points. To ensure that tension can be evenly balanced around the line and between the 2 points, all muscle fibers must be arranged in concentric cylinders with that line at their center. When a round muscle contracts, it closes like a fist around the blood vessels and traps lactic acid. For example, the bicep is a round muscle, and the pectoralis major (in the chest) and the deltoids (shoulder) are both made up of flat and round sections. All flat and round skeletal muscles, and their tendons, could become spastic at their attachments. Why? Because muscle attachments curve inward just before they attach to the bone, which in turn allows lactic acid to become trapped. The deeper muscle tissues are insensate; they lack pain-sensing nerve fibers. Any pain felt from a spasm is the result of some kind of irritation transmitted to superficial muscles. "Lactic acid is our villain. It is the cause of hypertonic spasm. Lactic acid is produced when an animal cell metabolizes sugar anaerobically—without using oxygen. Whenever our muscles are at work—and that's all the time—they produce lactic acid. The harder and more sustained the muscle activity, the greater the output of lactic acid." So, by learning how to focus attention to the specific muscles that, when contracted, create joint mobility, the body moves efficiently and the mind is given a concentration point for direction, a *dharana*.

In addition, when you train yourself to have an additional point of awareness upon the conscious relaxation of the antagonist, the stretching muscles, there is a deep relaxation reflex that occurs, promoting proper effort without stress. As an example, in the Cat Pose, when going into spine flexion and lifting the spine, if no attention is given to contracting the rectus abdominis muscle, the major muscle of trunk flexion, the movement of the back will not be full. Once you learn where the muscle is and how to focus your attention on a full contraction of the entire muscle, your lumbar and thoracic spinal regions will be given a full flexion motion. This movement can become even greater, although it is subtle, by an additional awareness that promotes conscious relaxation of the deep spinal muscles, the erector spinae.

In this manner, by learning functional anatomy, you will definitely increase your joint freedom, muscular stamina, concentration and capacity to relax. Movement results from muscles contracting through a specific pattern of motion to pull the bones in various directions to open or close the joints (see the following table). In any given movement, the forces involved include both the primary and secondary movers. The primary movers exert their contractile forces in a pattern corresponding to the line of their muscle fibers from the beginning tendon, called the origin, to the end-point tendon, called the insertion. The secondary movers exert their forces at an angle to the motion and are hence less efficient. In learning anatomy, it is helpful to learn the primary movers of joint action.

## Muscle Pairs and Their Corresponding Movements

| MUSCLE | MOVEMENT | ANTAGONIST | MOVEMENT |
|---|---|---|---|
| Sternocleidomastoid (SCM) | Lateral neck flexion, rotation | SCM on the opposite side | Opposite lateral flexion, rotation |
| Sternocleidomastoid | Neck flexion | Upper trapezius | Neck extension |
| Middle trapezius | Shoulder adduction, external rotation | Pectoralis major, serratus anterior | Shoulder abduction, internal rotation |
| Anterior deltoid | Shoulder flexion | Posterior deltoid | Shoulder extension |

*Cont'd...*

| MUSCLE | MOVEMENT | ANTAGONIST | MOVEMENT |
|---|---|---|---|
| Biceps brachii | Elbow flexion | Triceps brachii | Elbow extension |
| Flexor carpi radialis/ulnaris | Wrist flexion | Extensor carpi radialis longus | Wrist extension |
| Rectus abdominis | Spinal flexion | Erector spinae, latissimus longus | Spinal extension |
| Gluteus maximus | Hip extension | Psoas, rectus femoris | Hip flexion |
| Gluteus medius | Hip abduction | Adductors, gracilis | Hip adduction |
| Gluteus minimus, tensor fascia lata | Hip internal rotation | Psoas, external hip rotator group | Hip external rotation |
| Hamstrings | Knee flexion | Quadriceps | Knee extension |
| Gastronemus, Soleus | Ankle plantar flexion | Tibialis anterior | Ankle dorsiflexion |

## Summary

Muscle is the largest type of tissue in your body and is extremely malleable because it responds to the type, duration and intensity of exercise that we perform. Frequently exercised muscle tissue is in a constant state of remodeling, leading to increases in endurance, strength, flexibility and power.

## Bone Tissue

Bones are a dynamic living tissue that forms the body's structural framework. Bone mass is composed of organic and inorganic materials, including calcium salts and connective tissue, as well as cells and blood vessels within a calcium matrix. This combination gives bone a tensile strength near to that of steel; yet, it remains a medium of elasticity. By aligning the direction of the force of gravity along the major axis of the bones, we can access its strength in yoga postures.

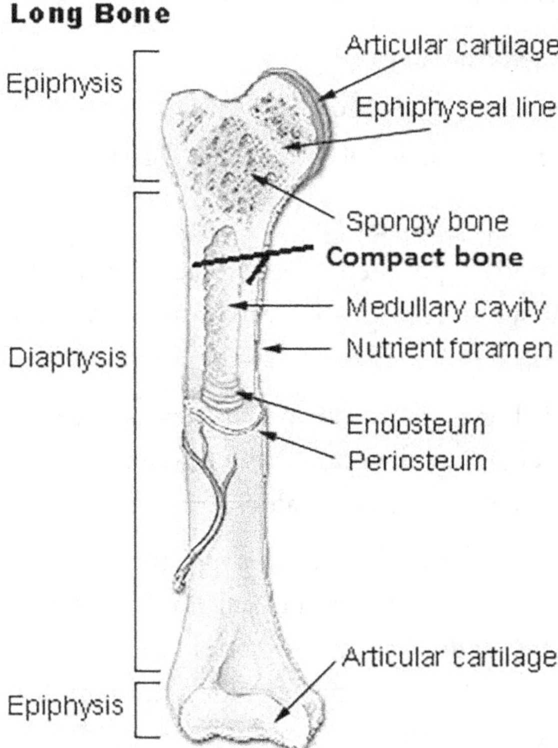



Bones are alive. They have blood supply. They have nerves running in and out of them. If they get bruised or hit hard, you feel it. The bone is constantly going through changes on a cellular level, as cells are created, broken down and rearranged based on the stresses they have to manage.

Bones are yet another varied formation of connective tissue in the body. A thick layer of connective tissue, called periosteum, surrounds the outer surface of bone. Inside the bone is the medullary cavity, which contains bone marrow. Along the inside of this cavity is another layer of connective tissue called the endo-osteum. In between these layers of connective tissue are the crystallized minerals that make our bones hard. Primarily, these minerals are calcium and phosphorus. Within them are the hollow areas that allow nerves and blood supply to move through the bones.

The skeletal system has 5 basic functions.

- It provides structure,
- It produces red blood cells,
- It stores minerals,
- It protects vital organs and
- It enables movement.

There are 3 types of bone cells:

1. Bone-building cells called osteoblasts,
2. Mature bone cells called osteocytes and
3. Cells that break down mature bone cells called osteoclast.

As bones are built, minerals are crystalized and built into the structure of the bone. If calcium or phosphorus is needed in the blood supply, then osteocytes may be broken down by osteoclasts to release these minerals into the blood supply. A similar mechanism allows bones to recreate their structure based on the stress placed on them. So, the skeletal system reacts to stress and stimuli placed on it.

Regular practice of yoga is beneficial to our bones because healthy stress is applied in a variety of unusual directions. This strengthens the bones, which remodel in response to stress by depositing layers of calcium into the bone matrix. Lack of healthy stress on bones weakens them.

Bones are also the body's reservoir of calcium, supporting a variety of physiological functions including muscle contraction. The concentration of calcium in the body is tightly regulated through a complex interplay of skeletal, endocrine and excretory functions. This involves feedback loops between the parathyroid gland, the kidneys, the intestines, the skin, the liver and the bones. Calcium absorption in the human gut is dependent on stable support of Vitamin D and estrogen balance. So, make sure to have adequate calcium intake on a daily basis. High calcium foods include millets, **dark leafy greens, cheese, low-fat milk** and **yogurt, bok choy**, fortified **tofu**, okra, **broccoli**, green beans, almonds and **fish canned** with their bones. The daily value (DV) for calcium is 1000mg.

## *Foods That Provide Vitamin D Include*

- Fatty fish like tuna, mackerel and salmon.
- Dairy products, orange juice, soy milk and cereals.
- Cheese.
- Egg yolks.

## *Estrogenic Foods*

- Dried fruits, especially dried apricots, dates and prunes, can help balance your estrogen levels in a big way.
- Flaxseed.
- Sesame Seeds.
- Chickpeas.
- Soya beans.
- Peas.
- Tempeh.
- Alfalfa Sprouts.

You can also use this list of estrogenic foods as a way to avoid foods high in estrogen if you have too much estrogen in your body.

Bone mass decreases in osteoporosis. This age-related decrease is associated with the loss of estrogen in post-menopausal women. Studies have demonstrated that resistance-type exercise maintains bone mass.

The bones of the skeleton link together at the joints and act as levers for the muscles that cross the joints. Consciously contracting and relaxing these skeletal muscles moves the body into various yoga postures.

Accordingly, it is reasonable to conclude that the various healthy stresses that yoga practice applies across the bones will aid in preventing osteoporosis.

## Joints

To take full advantage of our body's capabilities, we need to learn more about the anatomy of our joints. Where bones meet at a joint, they are tipped with cartilage that serves to cushion the meeting of bones in their movements. A joint capsule, a membrane containing synovial fluid that lubricates the surfaces to provide smooth movement, surrounds the joint. When healthy, the synovial fluid and cartilage allow for complete ease and freedom of motion without aches or pains. During normal motion, muscles contract on one side of the joint, while the antagonist muscle on the opposite side relaxes. Hence, half our muscular activity is created by tension. The other half is a simultaneous relaxation. Lack of either component will create lack of coordination. Muscular tension compresses the joint space.

When a person's nervous system has not learned to relax during motion, muscular tension can damage the cartilage or joint capsule. The signal that we are experiencing change begins with subtle messages like the feeling of being stiff. If ignored, these become feelings of tiredness, awkwardness, lack of coordination, then progress to aches, pains and disease.

Classical Yoga guidelines encourages us to seek positions in which we continually experience our body to be "comfortable and steady." The loss of comfort begins a spectrum from discomfort, to pain, to pathology. When we fail to listen to this message and make a change in how we experience our bodies, we move away from yoga. Each joint is a world of its own, with its own limitations according to its anatomical structure (Range of movement or ROM), specific functions, and structure that make it unique, relative to other joints. Problems can arise from several factors:

- We don't know where the joint is, so in order to move, we exert misdirected tension that accumulates in the muscle belly.
- We don't know how to minimize the tension involved in muscular action.
- We don't know what normal mobility is and when we are not in alignment during motion, detrimental stress arises.
- The sensations of being comfortable and steady in our bodies is lost.

The last is the most critical of all. For yoga to be effective, we must be conscious and aware of the differences between comfort and discomfort. Yet, consciousness is not enough. There must also be a discipline toward freedom from discomfort and disease. To practice yoga is to refine our awareness consistently over the span of a lifetime. We need to learn all of these factors to be free of joint pain.

By creating a healthy amount of joint space, working in alignment and training ourselves to minimize the tensions of muscular activity, movement can become so natural that we again enjoy the very best circulatory health. Freedom of the joints can provide for independent movement at each joint. Without this, the body may move unnecessarily in other joints. For instance, when you raise your right arm above your head, your left shoulder may rise, creating excessive stress around the neck. This creates a tremendous waste of energy and increases the wear and tear on tissues. Besides, it doesn't feel good to accumulate tension.

By learning to create relaxation, alignment and space during motion, you bring a transformation in your experience of living in the body home. To understand the mechanics of motion, you must be trained to feel your body in unfamiliar ways. Learning how to do yoga poses is not enough. The student of yoga also needs to learn how to feel himself. Teachers will ask, "What do you feel when you do yoga? Where do you feel the movement or the holding of a position?" They will also inform you about the correctness of this feeling. If you are feeling tension in a part of your body that should be relaxing, they will assist you to shift your effort to more beneficial areas. If the tension is appropriate, they will assist you in learning what that signal is as well. You will learn the difference between muscle and nerve sensation, strength and stretch sensations, good and bad pain.

This education of feelings is a natural part of the yoga class curriculum. Learning to listen to your body's messages can be taught by a good yoga teacher who gives you pauses during the instructions so you can sense and feel your way back into a proper relationship with your body's many parts. The body's mass is composed of 60 percent muscle and skeletal tissues. This is a tremendous amount, and the major portion of the body's signals come from sensors located in these tissues. While visual stimuli make the majority of our sensory input, the messages from muscles, joints and skin are also significant.

## Types of Joints

There are 6 types of synovial joints classified according to their function, shape or both.

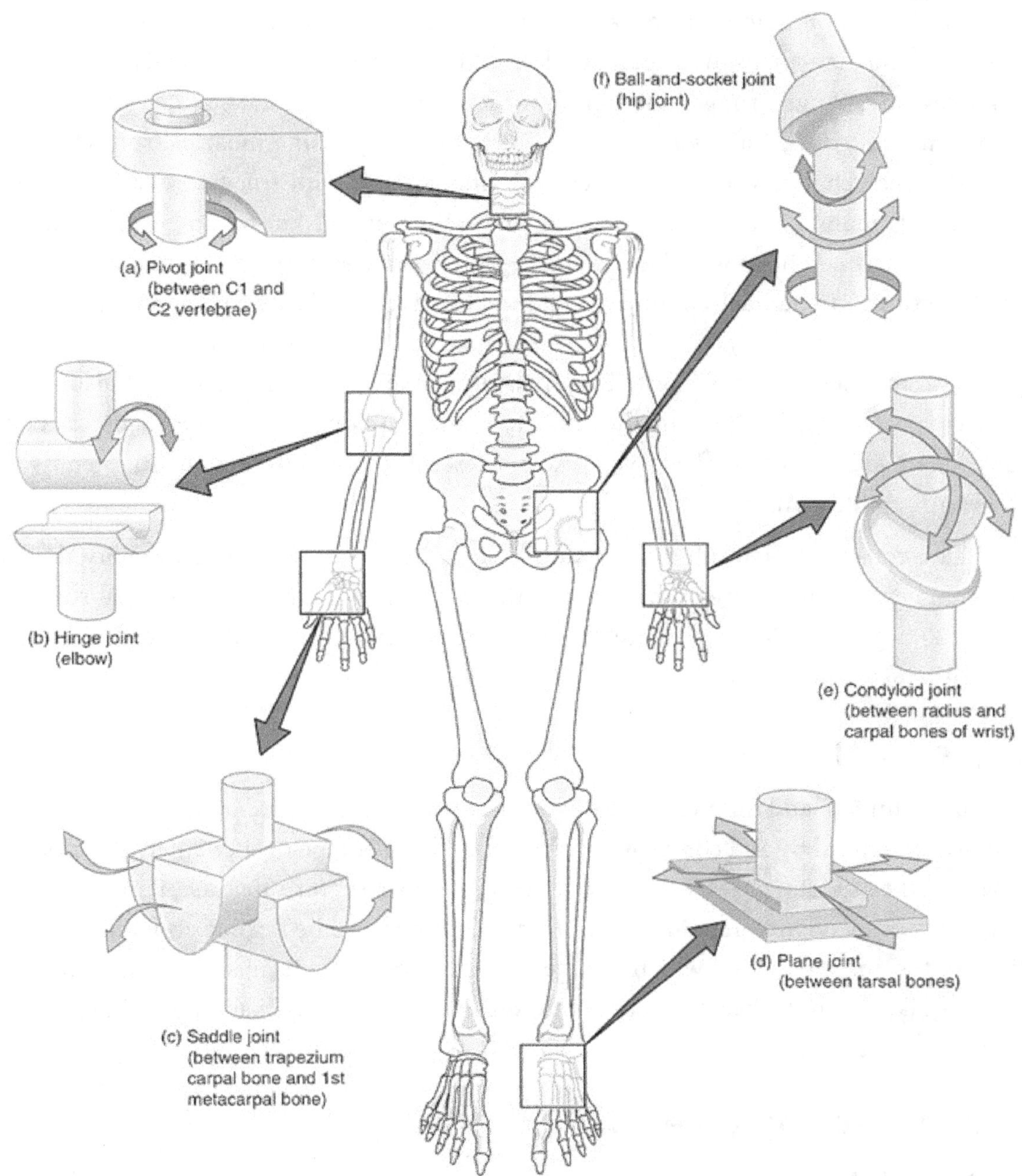



## *Joint Freedom*

Joint freedom is the ability of each joint to move freely through its full range of motion without cracking, muscular stress, discomfort or causing movement in the adjacent joints. It is not a common phenomenon, even in trained athletes or yogis and is dependent upon several factors. Among them are balances of muscle tone with elasticity and healthy connective tissue, which surrounds muscles to define their shape, keeps their muscular activity independent of adjacent muscles and serves to bind muscles to bones and keep healthy bones free of extraneous material (bone spurs and/or arthritis). The resulting flexibility varies from person to person according to several criteria—the activities we engage in (and how coordinated and balanced we are while active); our age; sex; weight; genetic postural imbalances; injuries; pain; body conditioning and our emotional state. For example, running makes hamstrings stronger and tighter, which in turn lessens our standing forward-bending (hip flexion) mobility. Continually running can prevent the opposing muscles from working freely. Over time, this may change your posture. Our optimal age for joint freedom is ages 3 to 5, but for some people, it is maintained into the preteen years. Women are known to be more flexible than men. You may have been born with knock-knees, which will lessen the distance you can open your legs (hip abduction). If you have asthma, you'll tend to have less ability to reverse the curve of your upper back (thoracic extension). When people are depressed, they tend to collapse forward, rounding the upper back and caving in the chest. This not only makes breathing shallow, it also tightens the chest muscles (pectorals), diminishing the capacity of the shoulders to be pulled backward (shoulder extension). There are many benefits to yoga. Yoga exercises that maintain your suppleness may be a factor in extending lifespan.

While I have consulted all the physical medical association standards of joint mobility, the standards set here are, in general, an average. I have found that increasing the range of external rotation of the hips by 10 to 20 degrees (to 55 or 65 degrees) is more beneficial to the health of the spinal column and longevity of hip joints.

# The Knee Joint

As we attempt to understand different joints of our body, we must explore in detail the knee joint. The knee is highly influenced by and connected to the joints above and below it, namely the foot and ankle joint below and the hip joint above. It is a very strong joint by structure, because a great amount of our body weight passes through it. In addition to strength, it must also be flexible enough to deal with the adaptations of the ankle and foot, which change shape and position. It must also adapt to the hip and its role as we walk. When the balance between these joints, their strength and flexibility goes away, the knee often receives the force.

## *Basic Anatomy of the Knee Joint*

Knee pain and dysfunction are almost as common as back pain. In India, sitting on the floor has been a way of life for a long time. Although this is slowly disappearing with Western influence, you will still see people squatting to carry out many household activities. And let's not forget the Eastern toilet: porcelain laid in the floor requiring that you squat to use it. With all this squatting and sitting down on the floor variations, hips and knees stay more flexible than others. Therefore, it is practically assumed that the Lotus pose can be done. Lotus variations are the norm in the culture in which yoga was created. So, it is important to understand all the components of the posture, work with them over time and let your lotus pose grow at its own pace.

The knee is one of the largest and most complex joints in the body. The knee joins the thigh bone (femur) to the shin bone (tibia). The smaller bone that runs alongside the tibia (fibula) and the kneecap (patella) are the other bones that make the knee joint.

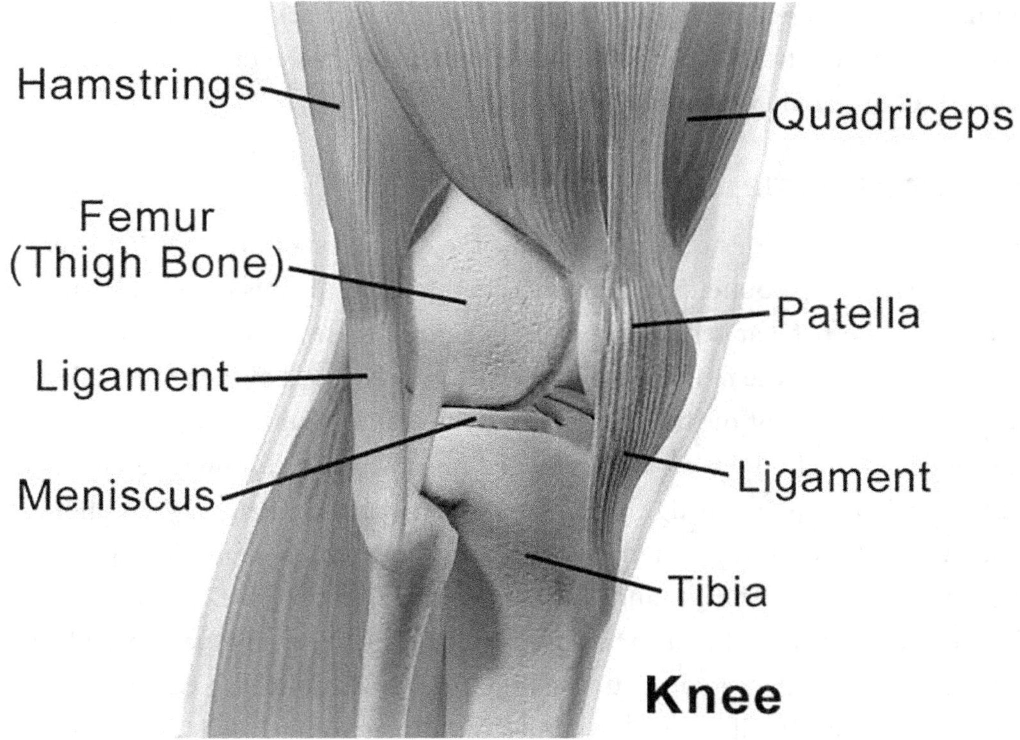



Tendons connect the knee bones to the leg muscles that move the knee joint. Ligaments join the knee bones and provide stability to the knee: The anterior cruciate ligament prevents the femur from sliding backward on the tibia (or the tibia sliding forward on the femur). The posterior cruciate ligament prevents the femur from sliding forward on the tibia (or the tibia from sliding backward on the femur). The medial and lateral collateral ligaments prevent the femur from sliding side to side. Two C-shaped pieces of cartilage called the medial and lateral menisci act as shock absorbers between the femur and tibia. Numerous bursae, or fluid-filled sacs, help the knee move smoothly.

## *The Meniscus*

The 2 bones that stand in end-to-end apposition to one another in the knee joints, the tibia and the femur can withstand the repetitive shocks of walking and running because they are well cushioned. The lower ends of the femurs (femoral condyles) and the upper ends of the tibias (tibial condyles) are covered with thick layers of articular hyaline cartilage that have a slippery surface for permitting flexion and extension. In addition, donut-shaped wafers of fibrocartilage, called the medial and lateral menisci (or medial and lateral semilunar cartilages), cushion the mating surfaces of the condyles. Torn menisci are difficult to treat because they have lost their blood supply by the time we reach our mid-20s, and if they are damaged after that time, usually in dance or athletics, they are essentially irreparable. This is why "torn cartilages" are greeted so apprehensively by adult athletes.

The menisci move freely during the course of flexion. This is not ordinarily a problem because we assume that they will come back into their home position when the knee joint is subsequently extended. But that does not always happen, and if it doesn't, the menisci can get crushed by the opposing condyles. This might happen when you kick a ball or start to get up from a squatting position, and if you ever encounter unusual resistance to extension under such circumstances, carefully sit down and massage the knee before you try to straighten it. If you crush the menisci the only remedy may be trimming them surgically, if not removing them outright.

## The Patella and Bursae

The main role of the patella, or kneecap, is to make the extension of the knee joint more efficient. It is a sesamoid bone, that is, a bone that is inserted in a tendon, in this case between the quadriceps femoris tendon and the patellar tendon. During flexion, it slides down the intercondylar notch, a deep vertical gutter between the femoral condyles (the articular end of the femur); during extension, it acts like a pulley on the front of the knee. The patella is important in any activity where the knee supports the weight of the body in a partially flexed position. You can imagine how useful it is in a standing lunge or when you are rising from a half squat with a barbell on your shoulders. In these activities, your entire body is supported by the quadriceps femoris muscles, quadriceps tendons, patella and patellar tendons. The up and down movement of the patella is made possible by the suprapatellar bursa, a lubricant-filled sack that is situated between the patella and the underlying tissues. Bursae are common accessories to many joints whose attaching tendons move in relation to their underlying tissues. If adhesions resulting from disease, injury or inactivity develop within a bursa, the tendon can no longer slip back and forth easily. And this, in the case of the suprapatellar bursa, is one of the commonest causes of a "stiff knee" following traumatic injury. A circular problem may develop—you can't flex the knee because of the injury, the bursa develops adhesions and the adhesions further inhibit mobility. Again, the practical concern in hatha yoga is with old injuries. If they flare up, students so affected should be cautioned not to do any postures that stress the knees until the problem is resolved.

## Synovial Fluid

Synovial fluid is the slippery fluid that fills most of the body's joints. All joints occur where 2 separate bones intersect or overlap, but there are a few that don't contain synovial fluid and have very limited movement, including the intervertebral (between the vertebrae) discs and the 2 sacroiliac joints on the back of the pelvis. The rest are synovial joints, which are freely moveable and need a system that cushions the ends of the bones, allowing them to glide over each other without friction. This system consists of hyaline cartilage, the smooth, whitish covering on the ends of the bones, and the synovial fluid, which fills the space between the cartilage surfaces and facilitates smooth, painless movement between bones. This clear, slightly viscous fluid is also important because it delivers nutrients and oxygen to the hyaline cartilage, which—unlike most body tissues—doesn't have its own blood supply. Any joint movement helps circulate the synovial fluid, which feeds the cartilage; practicing yoga poses, therefore, helps keep the cartilage well nourished.

When my students are feeling warm and good and happy after a class, I jokingly ask if they feel like they've just had a tune-up and oil change. In fact, while yoga doesn't change any fluids, it does do a wonderful job of moving fluids around in your body. Your blood circulates in your arteries and veins and your lymph flows through the spaces around all your cells; both fluids can be cleansed of metabolic by-products and your blood replenished with oxygen and nutrients. Yoga also helps circulate the synovial fluid inside your joints.

Each synovial joint has a fibrous capsule surrounding the joint, which helps hold the bones together, along with the ligaments (which join bone to bone) and tendons (which join muscle to bone). The joint capsule is lined by the synovial membrane, which manufactures the synovial fluid. Your body automatically produces the necessary amount of this lubricating fluid. Although the idea that yoga stimulates production of synovial fluid creates a lovely image, there actually isn't any time when the well runs dry.

## Inflammation of the Knee Joint: When Too Much Is Too Much

In fact, the only problem with amount of fluid occurs when there is too much. This problem is part of the inflammatory process, which is defined by the presence of swelling, pain, redness and heat. Inflammation is the body's response to injury, as well as part of the process of arthritis, which includes the wearing of hyaline cartilage. (In more advanced cases of osteoarthritis—the wear-and-tear arthritis commonly associated with old age—and in rheumatoid arthritis—the autoimmune disease in which the body attacks its own joint tissues—the synovial membrane also becomes painfully inflamed, and the cartilage can wear away until bone rests painfully on bone.)

Because increased synovial fluid production—we see it as swelling—is associated with injury and inflammation, you don't want your yoga practice to stimulate this production. In fact, we as teachers should encourage students to practice in such a way that, over the months and years, their joints become healthier and stronger and they avoid strain and injury. One of the best ways to avoid joint damage is to teach students to pay attention to any pain in or directly around a joint, and to modify or change the alignment of the pose to eliminate that pain. Pain in or around a joint means: you are overstretching connective tissue, such as tendons and ligaments (which are designed to stabilize joints and will cause a joint to become hypermobile if overstretched) or you are compressing the joint surfaces, which can contribute to arthritis. So "no joint pain" should be your teaching rule. Leave the work on joints to trained healthcare professionals who know whether, and precisely how, to improve joint mobility without damaging the joint's cartilage or support system.

On the other hand, what should a teacher do if a student arrives in class with an already inflamed joint? A common example is a sprained ankle, which is painful, swollen, hot and probably red. Ankle ligaments are often violently overstretched by stepping in a hole or slipping off a high heel, but any joint can become inflamed by damage to a ligament or tendon. Common examples are tears, which are often associated with accidents and athletic activities, and overworking a joint beyond its current level of condition. Overworking a joint to the point of inflammation can occur while doing yoga, perhaps by repetitively practicing a pose in incorrect alignment and thereby putting strain on ligaments or tendons. Also, seriously deconditioned or even atrophied shoulder muscles, for example, can easily be overworked by even a few Sun Salutations. And arthritis, of course, provides joint conditions that are easily provoked into inflammation.

## *Responding to inflammation*

The bottom line here is that an inflamed joint should never be pushed, stretched into pain, or worked vigorously, because the risk of increasing or prolonging the inflammation is great. It's much better to train your students to respond to the inflammation in a way that promotes health. Use the example of a sprained ankle to guide your problem solving. A sprained ankle is usually stabilized with a wraparound bandage, brace or, in severe cases, even a cast. These stabilizers prevent movement, allowing the strained tissues to heal without disturbance. But if, instead, you move and stretch and work an inflamed joint, you'll likely cause repetitive micro trauma, which disrupts the healing process and may actually cause more damage.

So, when dealing with inflammation, encourage your student to work vigorously on other parts of the body and to choose poses that keep the inflamed joint relatively quiet until the pain and swelling have receded significantly. This is not to say you shouldn't move the joint at all; mild, unforced movements help the healing process by circulating the blood to ligaments, tendons and muscles and by circulating synovial fluid to hyaline cartilage. However, if the inflammation or pain is severe or the problem shows no improvement or is even getting worse, urge your student to see a healthcare provider to evaluate the problem, run necessary tests and prescribe a treatment plan.

## **Muscles around the Knee Joint**

The following muscles all act at the knee joint to flex, extend and rotate the knee:

- Extensors: quadriceps femoris (rectus femoris, vastus medialis, vastus lateralis and vastus intermedius); tensor fasciae latae
- Flexors: hamstrings (biceps femoris, semitendinosus and semimembranosus); popliteus; gracilis; sartorius
- Internal (medial) rotators: semimembranosus; popliteus; pes anserinus (semitendinosus, gracilis, sartorius)
- External (lateral) rotators: biceps femoris (possibly aided by the tensor fasciae latae as the knee moves into flexion)

## **Pain in the Knee Joint?**

Knee joint pain management is high on the priority list for every yoga student and teacher. During every consultation, anatomy classes and workshops I conduct, people will ask for knee joint pain management in asana practice.

The ideal image of yoga in most of the world is someone sitting in the Lotus Pose. Therefore, the Lotus Pose becomes a measuring stick for a person's yoga practice. Approximately 80 percent of people complain about knee joint pain in the Lotus Pose where the leg is flexed and rotated. They experience pain on the medial side of the knee joint.

Around 10-15 percent of people complain about pain on the lateral side of the knee joint. However, some people complain about pain through the centerline of their knee around the knee cap. All these 3 areas express stress in the knee in different ways.

The Lotus Pose requires 2 movements, which, when combined, put the most amount of pressure on the medial meniscus. These 2 movements are

- flexion of the knee and
- medial rotation of the tibia.

Both the femur and tibia have to rotate externally. If the tibia doesn't have enough outward rotation, there could still be enough in the hip to make up for it, or vice versa.

If both femur and tibia lack the ability to rotate externally, we will end up moving in internal rotation which can put pressure on the medial meniscus. When we combine this with a flexed knee, as in the Lotus Pose, we end up with even more pressure on the medial meniscus. On top of it, if the hips are tight, it is common to feel pressure in the knee. Yoga practice is unlikely to damage the knees as asanas do not impact the knee unlike in sports. However, if there exists a previous problem like bone chip, tendinitis or meniscus tear, repeated bending, folding, stretching or twisting the knees in yoga could irritate the nerves around the knee cap and also overstretch the tendons.

There are other structures in the area that can get inflamed or irritated and cause pain on the inside of the knee. For instance, the medial collateral ligament and various muscles crossing the inside of the knee, and even the joint capsule itself, can get compressed and irritated.

There are 2 ways of dealing with this:

The first is an immediate response—the moment you feel the sensation of pain, place one hand on your thigh near your knee and the other on your calf muscle and then try rotating both of them externally, as if you are creating space between the ends of the 2 bones rotationally. You could also prop the knee higher with a block to see if that alleviates the pressure or pain.

Some people complain about pain on the inside of the knee joint and experience a "pop" in the lotus position. Swelling in the back of the knee and sometimes a regular clicking sound is followed by the "pop" sound. It is also possible that the knee will lock intermittently after the first "pop" sound occurs. All of these are the classic signs and symptoms of the meniscus tear. The best way to confirm if the meniscus has torn out is to consult a doctor.

The long-term solution for all these problems of the knee joint is to lengthen the tissues in the hip that are resisting external rotation of the joint.

## *Care*

- Holding the asana without the knowledge of proper alignment results in one of the bones or muscles being slightly out of alignment. This could cause physical stress due to an uneven distribution of weight which sometimes leads to a slight shift in the position of the knee cap, making the knee region prone to injuries.
- Flat feet or fallen arch is another condition which could cause knee pain.
- When the muscles along the thighs are not rotated properly while constructing an asana, it could lead to pain in the knees. It is a common oversight by many yoga practitioners. We should pay

attention to the IT band that runs along the length of the thighs on its sides. It is very common in runners and weight lifters to have tight hip muscles attached to this IT band, creating tension in the along the band. In these circumstances, some asanas could cause the tissues to thicken and bind, which pulls the knee and causes pain.

The following asanas help strengthen the area. These should not be practiced if the area is already injured or is in the process of healing.

**Standing asanas -**

Tadasana

Santulasana

Prasarita padottanasana (keep the knees slightly bend)

**Floor asanas -**

Setu Bandhasana

Gomukhasana

Akarna dhanurasana

Shalabhasana

Paschimottanasana

Urdhva mukha paschimottanasana

Halasana

## Knee Conditions

Chondro-malacia patella (also called patella-femoral syndrome): Irritation of the cartilage on the underside of the kneecap (patella), causing knee pain. This is a common cause of knee pain in young people.

Knee osteoarthritis: Osteoarthritis is the most common form of arthritis, and often affects the knees. Caused by aging and wear and tear of cartilage, osteoarthritis symptoms may include knee pain, stiffness and swelling.

Knee effusion: Fluid buildup inside the knee, usually from inflammation. Any form of arthritis or injury may cause a knee effusion.

Meniscal tear: Damage to a meniscus, the cartilage that cushions the knee, often occurs with twisting the knee. Large tears may cause the knee to lock.

ACL (anterior cruciate ligament) strain or tear: The ACL is responsible for a large part of the knee's stability. An ACL tear often leads to the knee "giving out," and may require surgical repair.

PCL (posterior cruciate ligament) strain or tear: PCL tears can cause pain, swelling and knee instability. These injuries are less common than ACL tears, and physical therapy (rather than surgery) is usually the best option.

MCL (medial collateral ligament) strain or tear: This injury may cause pain and possible instability to the inner side of the knee.

Patellar subluxation: The kneecap slides abnormally or dislocates along the thigh bone during activity, resulting in pain around the kneecap.

Patellar tendonitis: Inflammation of the tendon connecting the kneecap (patella) to the shin bone. This occurs mostly in athletes from repeated jumping.

Knee bursitis: Pain, swelling and warmth in any of the bursae of the knee. Bursitis often occurs from overuse or injury.

Baker's cyst: Collection of fluid in the back of the knee. Baker's cysts usually develop from a persistent effusion as in conditions such as arthritis.

Rheumatoid arthritis: An autoimmune condition that can cause arthritis in any joint, including the knees. If untreated, rheumatoid arthritis can cause permanent joint damage.

Gout: A form of arthritis caused by buildup of uric acid crystals in a joint. The knees may be affected, causing episodes of severe pain and swelling.

Pseudogout: A form of arthritis similar to gout, caused by calcium pyrophosphate crystals depositing in the knee or other joints.

Septic arthritis: Bacterial infection inside the knee can cause inflammation, pain, swelling and difficulty moving the knee. Although uncommon, septic arthritis is a serious condition that usually gets worse quickly without treatment.

## *Minor Knee Problems*

What can be done to prevent and resolve minor knee problems? The answer is simple—regular and prolonged muscular tension applied to the extended knee joint. Under such circumstances, all parts of the joint fit together perfectly, allowing it to withstand intense isometric contraction of the surrounding muscles. If you have knee pain which is not due to serious internal injuries, the following series of standing postures can be highly therapeutic. Keep the feet parallel and as widely separated as possible while holding the thigh muscles firmly, especially the adductors. Extending the knees fully is fine provided you do not hyperextend them beyond 180° and provided you hold tension in the hamstrings as well as the quadriceps femoris muscles. Holding a firm base with isometric tension is the whole point of this series. Twist right, then left, then face the front; in each direction bend forward and backward, holding each position for 2–7 breaths (5–30 seconds). That's 6 combinations. Hold the arms in various positions—elbows grasped behind the back; arms and forearms stretched laterally; hands in a prayer position behind the back; arms overhead with forearms behind the head and catching the elbows; hands interlocked behind the back and pulled to the rear; arms in a cow-face position first one way and then the other; and hands on the hips. That makes 6 times 8, which equals 48 poses. Start modestly, doing the postures only 5 minutes a day, and then gradually increase your commitment. If you spend 15 minutes a day on this series, you cannot help but strengthen the muscles that insert around the knee and place a healthy stress on the capsule of the knee joint, as well as on its associated tendons and ligaments. And this works wonders. After a few months of regular practice, the connective tissues of the joint will have gained enough strength and integrity, at least in the absence of serious medical problems, to withstand not only reasonable stresses on the knees in flexed positions, but also the stresses of sitting in cross-legged meditative postures.

## Psychological Associations

The knees are a symbol of inner determination and pride; the knees are also a symbol of willingness to bend to the flow of life, being willing to give yourself to your deepest Self without resistance, allowing yourself to move along the path of true evolution, without stubbornly holding on to false or outer values which could block that unfolding. In the knees lie the power to defend yourself and not let others push you, the strength that radiates your confidence. The knees allow you to kneel down to your deepest values as a divine being, honoring and respecting yourself and others, being flexible and open to the world. So, please take care of your knee joint by practicing the following set of knee joint strengthening exercises.

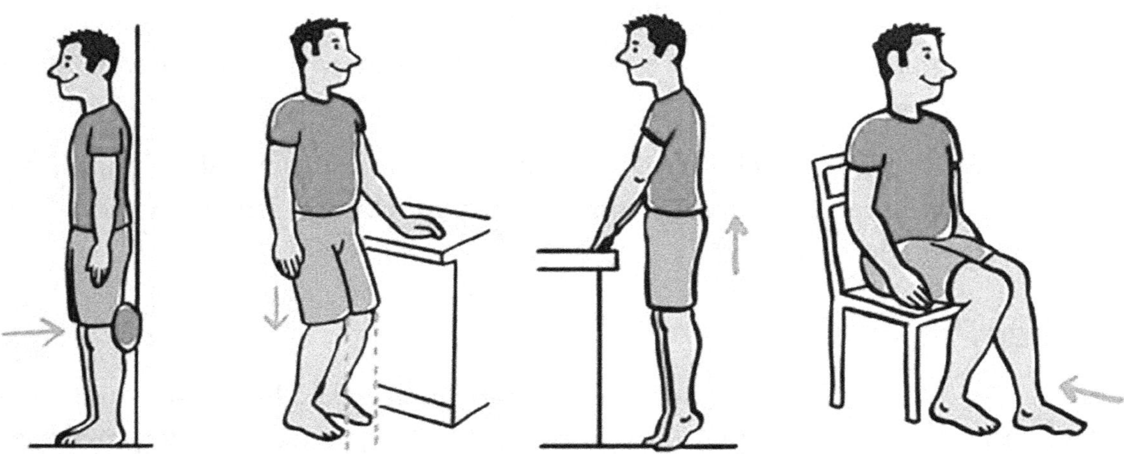

# The Hip Joint

The hip joint is an extremely moveable, ball and socket synovial joint, formed by an articulation between the pelvic acetabulum and the head of the femur.

It forms a connection from the lower limb to the pelvic girdle, and thus is designed for stability and weight-bearing, rather than a large range of movement.

Now, we shall look at the anatomy of the hip joint, its articulating surfaces, ligaments and neurovascular supply.

## The Structure of the Hip Joint

### Articulating Surfaces

The hip joint consists of an articulation between the head of the femur and the acetabulum of the pelvis.

The acetabulum is a cup-like depression located on the infero-lateral aspect of the pelvis. Its cavity is deepened by the presence of a fibro-cartilaginous collar—the acetabular labrum. The head of the femur is hemispherical and fits completely into the concavity of the acetabulum.

Both the acetabulum and head of femur are covered in articular cartilage, which is thicker at the weight-bearing places.

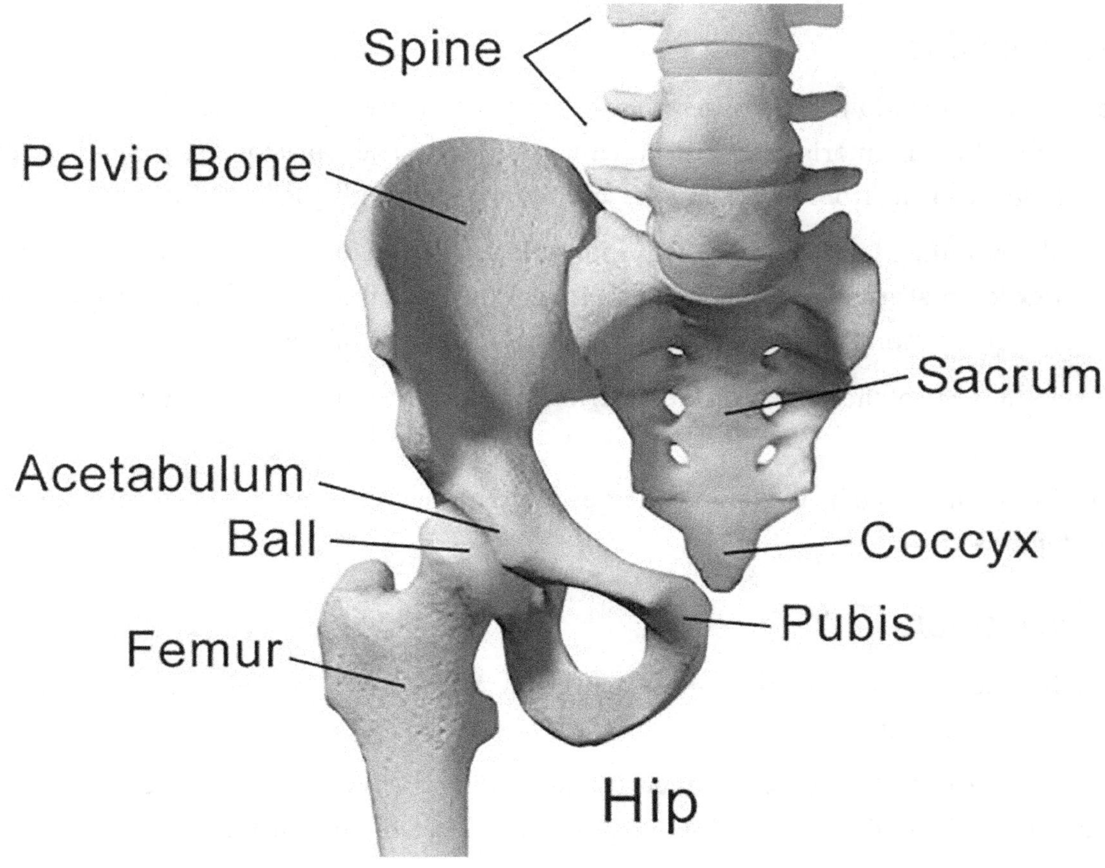


## Ligaments

The ligaments of the hip joint act to increase stability. They can be divided into 2 groups—intra-capsular and extra-capsular.

## Intra-Capsular

The only intra-capsular ligament is the one at the head of the femur. It is a relatively small structure, which runs from the acetabular fossa to the fovea of the femur. It encloses a branch of the obturator artery (artery at the head of the femur), a minor source of arterial supply to the hip joint.

## Extra-Capsular

There are 3 main extra-capsular ligaments, continuous with the outer surface of the hip joint capsule:

- Ilio-femoral ligament, which spans the area between the anterior inferior iliac spine and the intertrochanteric line of the femur. It has a 'Y' shaped appearance and prevents hyperextension of the hip joint.
- Pubo-femoral, which spans the area between the superior pubic rami and the intertrochanteric line of the femur. It has a triangular shape, and prevents excessive abduction and extension.

- Ischio-femoral, which spans the area between the body of the ischium and the greater trochanter of the femur. It has a spiral orientation and prevents excessive extension.

## Neurovascular Supply

The arterial supply to the hip joint is largely via the medial and lateral circumflex femoral arteries— branches of the profunda femoris artery (deep femoral artery). They anastomose at the base of the femoral neck to form a ring, from which smaller arteries arise to supply the hip joint itself.

The medial circumflex femoral artery is responsible for the majority of the arterial supply (the lateral circumflex femoral artery has to penetrate through the thick ilio-femoral ligament). Damage to the medial circumflex femoral artery can result in avascular necrosis of the femoral head.

The artery at the head of the femur and the superior/inferior gluteal arteries provide some additional supply.

The hip joint is innervated by the femoral nerve, obturator nerve, superior gluteal nerve and nerve to quadratus femoris.

## Stabilizing Factors

The primary function of the hip joint is to bear weight. There are a number of factors that act to increase stability of the joint.

The first structure is the acetabulum. It is deep, and encompasses nearly all of the head of the femur. This decreases the probability of the head slipping out of the acetabulum (dislocation).

There is a fibro-cartilaginous collar around the acetabulum that increases its depth, known as the acetabular labrum. The increase in depth provides a larger articular surface, further improving the stability of the joint.

The ilio-femoral, pubo-femoral and ischio-femoral ligaments are very strong, and along with the thickened joint capsule, provide a large degree of stability. These ligaments have a unique spiral orientation; this causes them to become tighter when the joint is extended.

In addition, the muscles and ligaments work in a reciprocal fashion at the hip joint:

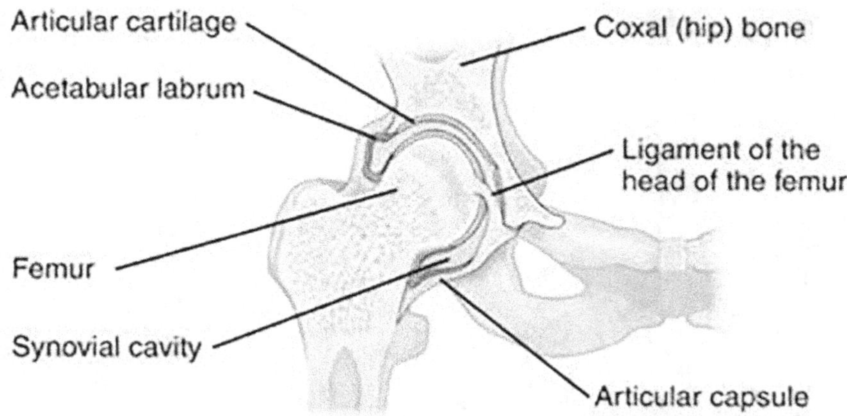


(a) Frontal section through the right hip joint

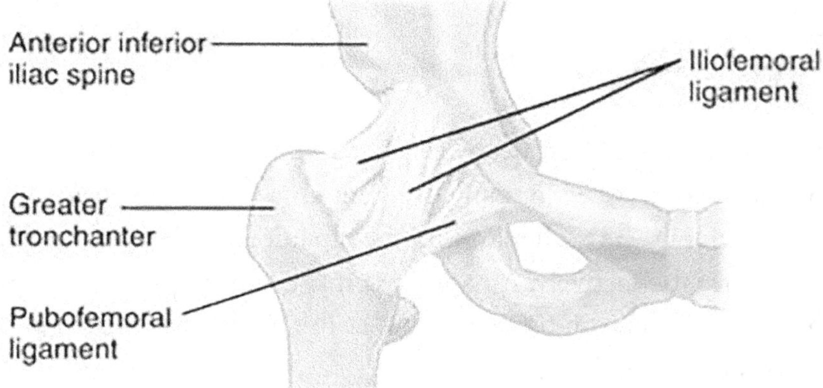


(b) Anterior view of right hip joint, capsule in place

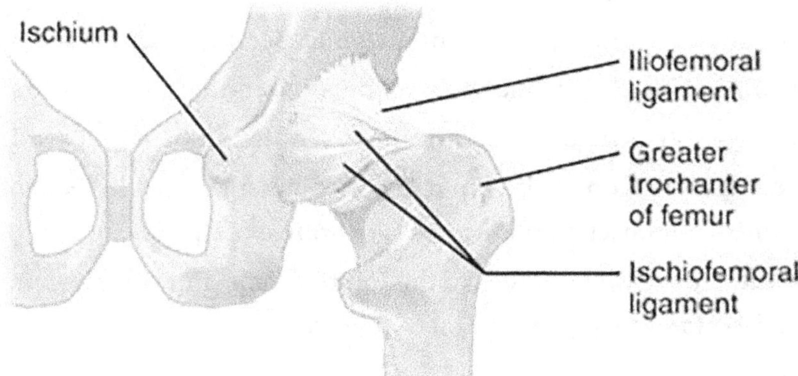


(c) Posterior view of right hip joint, capsule in place

Anteriorly, where the ligaments are strongest, the medial flexors (located anteriorly) are fewer and weaker.

Posteriorly, where the ligaments are weakest, the medial rotators are greater in number and stronger—they effectively "pull" the head of the femur into the acetabulum.

## *Movements and muscles*

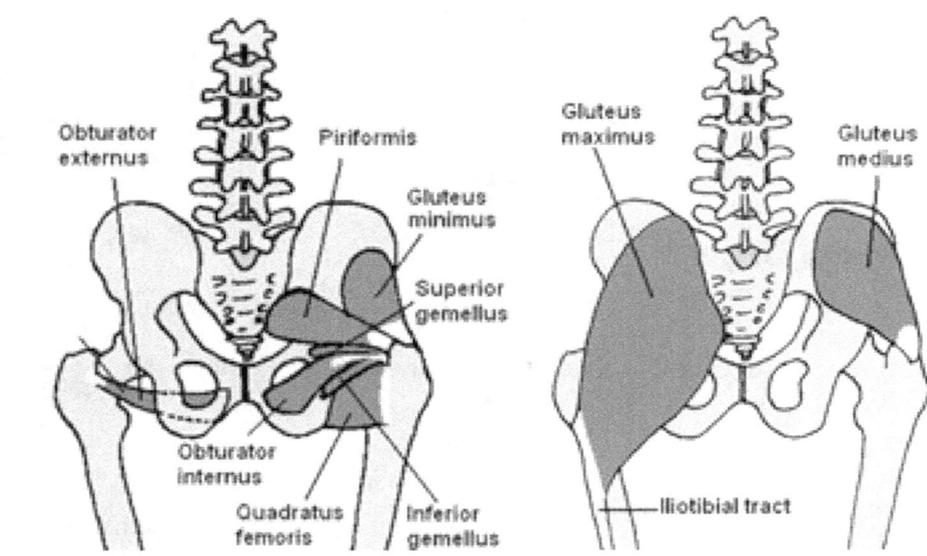


The hip joint is a multi-axial joint. This means that it can be moved in more than one axis. With a joint that has the possibility to move at so many different angles, we must have muscles that can pull the femur in all these directions. The tissues around the hip joint attach to and cross the hip joint at all the angles necessary to move it effectively. Any of these muscles, if tight, can also limit the hip's range of movement. The movements that can be carried out at the hip joint are listed below, along with the principal muscles responsible for each action:

- Flexion—iliopsoas, rectus femoris and sartorius
- Extension—gluteus maximus, semimembranosus, semitendinosus and biceps femoris
- Abduction—gluteus medius, gluteus minimus and the deep gluteals (piriformis, gemelli, etc.)
- Adduction—adductors longus, brevis and magnus, pectineus and gracillis
- Lateral rotation—biceps femoris, gluteus maximus and the deep gluteals (piriformis, gemelli, etc.)
- Medial rotation—gluteus medius and minimus, semitendinosus and semimembranosus

  The degree to which flexion at the hip can occur depends on whether the knee is flexed; this relaxes the hamstring muscles and increases the range of flexion.

  Extension at the hip joint is limited by the joint capsule and the ilio-femoral ligament. These structures become taut during extension to limit further movement.

# The Pelvis

The pelvic girdle is a ring-like structure, located in the lower part of the trunk. It connects the axial skeleton to the lower limbs.

In Latin, pelvis means "large bowl." The pelvis is not completely fused together until puberty. This is why we talk about 3 bones even though the pelvis looks like it is made of just one.

Now, we shall look at the structures of the pelvis, its functions and the applied anatomy.

## Structure of the Pelvic Girdle

The bony pelvis consists of the 2 hip bones (also known as innominate or pelvic bones), **sacrum** and **coccyx**.

There are 4 articulations within the pelvis:

- **Sacroiliac Joints (x2)**—between the ilium of the hip bones and the sacrum
- **Sacrococcygeal symphysis**—between the sacrum and the coccyx
- **Pubic symphysis**—between the pubis bodies of the 2 hip bones

## The Pelvic Girdle

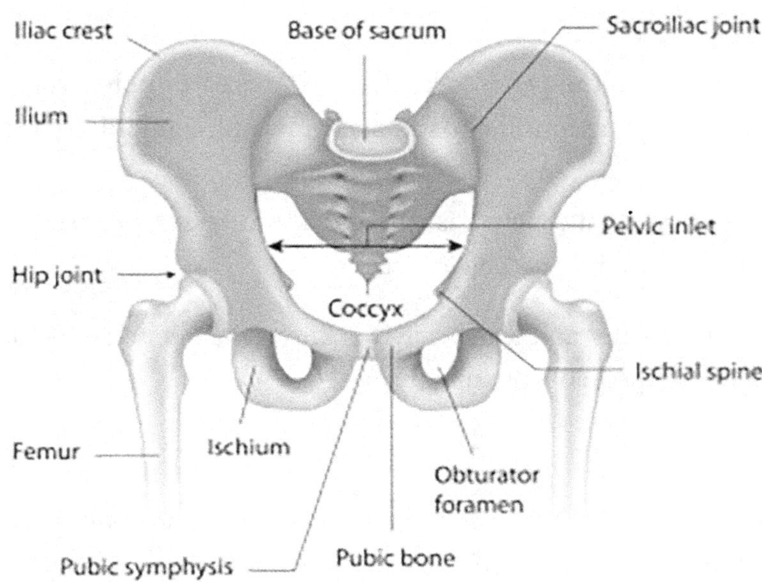


Ligaments attach the lateral border of the sacrum to various bony landmarks on the bony pelvis to aid **stability**.

## Functions of the Pelvis

The strong and rigid pelvis is adapted to serve numerous roles in the human body. The main functions being:

- **Transfer of weight** from the upper axial skeleton to the lower appendicular components of the skeleton, especially during movement.
- **Attachment** for several muscles and ligaments used in locomotion.
- **Containing and protecting** the abdomino-pelvic and pelvic viscera.

## The Greater and Lesser Pelvis

The osteology of the pelvic girdle allows the pelvic region to be divided into 2:

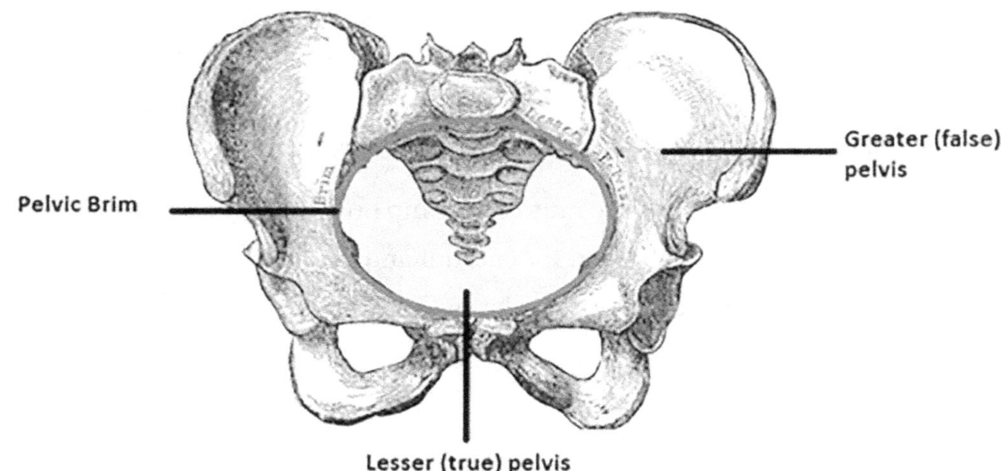


- The superior portion of the pelvis is known as the **greater pelvis** (or false pelvis). It provides support for the lower abdominal viscera (ileum and sigmoid colon) and has no obstetric relevance.
- The inferior portion of the pelvis is known as the **lesser pelvis** (or "true" pelvis). Within this reside the pelvic cavity and pelvic viscera.

The junction between the greater and lesser pelvis is known as the **pelvic inlet**. The outer bony edges of the pelvic inlet are called the **pelvic brim**.

## Pelvic Inlet

The pelvic inlet marks the boundary between the greater pelvis and lesser pelvis. Its size is defined by its edge, the **pelvic brim**.

The borders of the pelvic inlet:

- **Posterior**: the sacral promontory (the superior portion of the sacrum).
- **Lateral**: the arcuate line on the inner surface of the ilium and the pectineal line on the superior ramus.
- **Anterior**: the pubic symphysis.

The pelvic inlet determines the size and shape of the birth canal, with the prominent ridges, key areas of muscle and ligament attachment.

Some alternative descriptive terminology can be used in describing the pelvic inlet:

1. **Linea Terminalis:** refers to the combined pectineal line, arcuate line and sacral promontory.
2. **Iliopectineal line:** refers to the combined arcuate and pectineal lines.

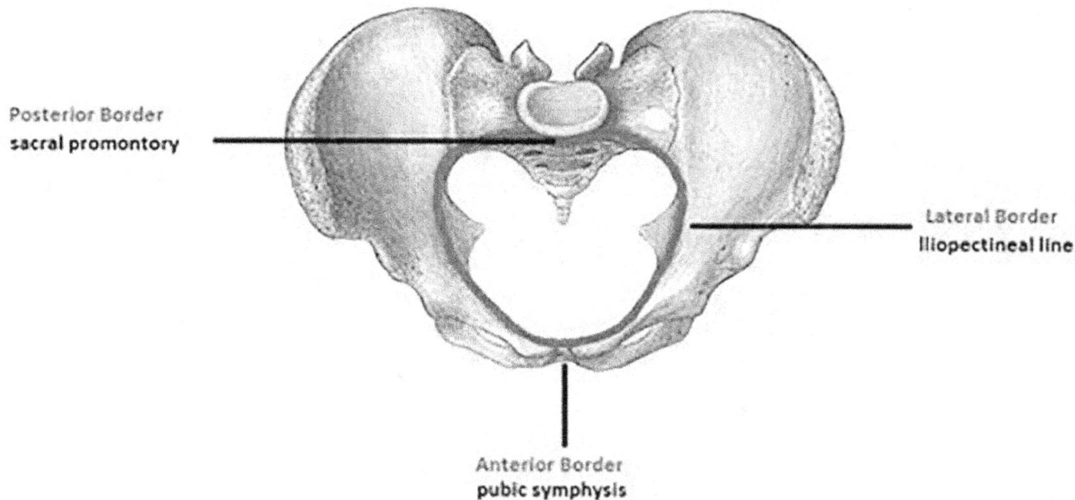


## Pelvic Outlet

The pelvic outlet is located at the end of the lesser pelvis and the beginning of the pelvic wall.

Its borders are:

- **Posterior**: the tip of the coccyx.
- **Lateral**: the ischial tuberosities and the inferior margin of the sacrotuberous ligament.
- **Anterior**: the pubic arch (the inferior border of the ischio-pubic rami).

The angle beneath the pubic arch is known as the **sub-pubic angle** and is of a greater size in women.

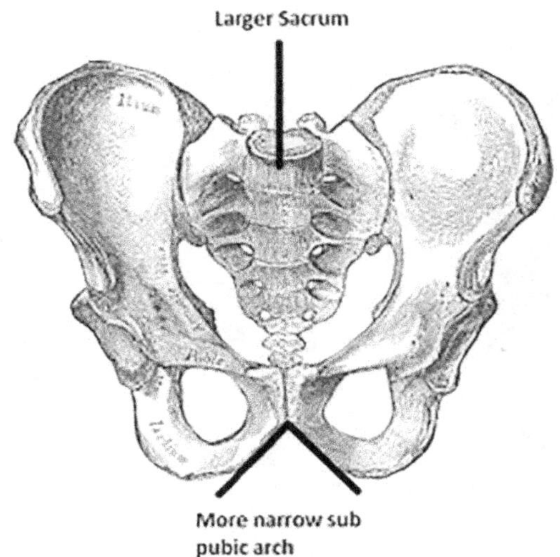

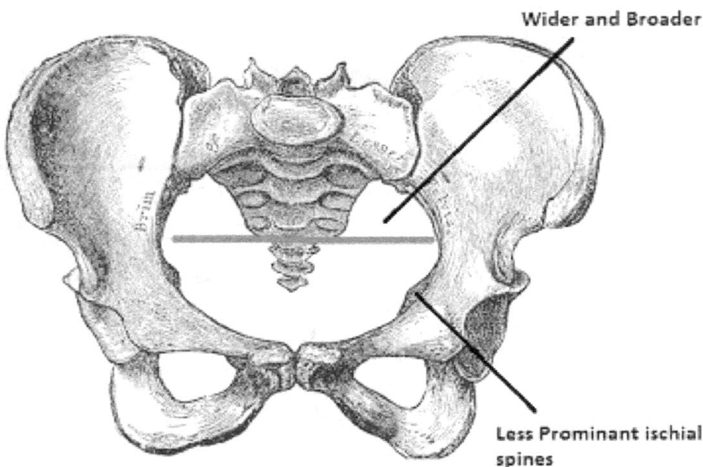



**Clinical relevance:** assessment of the female bony pelvis The lesser pelvis is the bony canal through which the fetus has to pass during childbirth. It is, therefore, of great importance to determine the diameter of this canal and thereby the childbearing capacity of the mother.

The diameter can be determined by a pelvic examination or radiographically. There are 2 measurements that are of importance:

## Obstetric Conjugate

To determine the narrowest fixed distance that the fetus would have to negotiate, the minimum antero-posterior diameter of the pelvic inlet is measured. This distance is between the sacral promontory and the midpoint of the pubic symphysis (where the pubic bone is thickest) and is known as the obstetric conjugate.

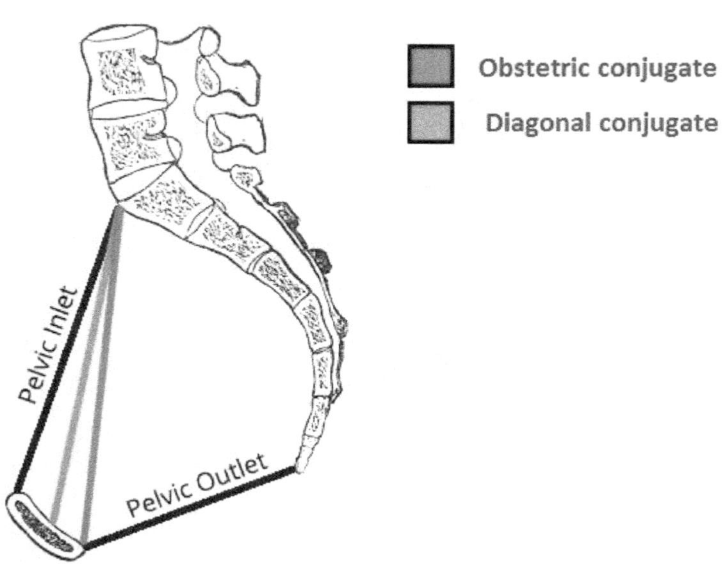

## Diagonal Conjugate

The diagonal conjugate is the alternative, measuring from the inferior border of the pubic symphysis to the sacral promontory and can be measured manually via the vagina.

## Sacroiliac Flexibility

Sacroiliac flexibility has until now been overlooked by those who write manuals on exercise and flexibility, and the terms nutation and counternutation are rarely encountered. This is not surprising since sacroiliac movements are limited to only 5–10° (except during the end stages of pregnancy), and these are overshadowed by the grosser movements of the spine and pelvis as a whole. Although the range of sacroiliac movements is narrow, however, healthy and mobile sacroiliac joints make for safer, sharper postures. Indeed, the proper execution and full expression of backward bending, forward bending and seated meditation postures presupposes the ability to establish nutation and counternutation at will. Because the concepts are unfamiliar and complex, some reiteration and review is in order. First, recall where the movements take place. They're not spinal movements (as happen at intervertebral discs and other joints in the spine), and they're not movements at the hip joints (as happen at the acetabula between the pelvic bones and the femurs). Rather, they are literally the only movements permitted between the axial skeleton and the appendicular skeleton for the lower extremities. And they are subtle: think of movements within the pelvis itself. If you want to understand the concepts, you will have to both think the movements through intellectually and appraise them experientially, and you have to do this while envisioning them not only in isolation but within larger bending gestures that involve the spine and the hip joints. These are not minor challenges.

## Nutation in Forward Bends

For both intermediate and advanced students, establishing nutation as a first priority in forward bends can be summed up easily: while maintaining the arched-forward lordosis in the lumbar region and while keeping the iliacus components of the iliopsoas complex relaxed, create a selective pull in the psoas muscles. You will sense little external movement, but the psoas muscles pull sharply forward on the lumbar region, and this, in turn, pulls the promontory of the sacrum forward, which favors nutation. The ilia are left behind and pulled medially by default as a result of keeping the iliacus muscles relaxed. Although not ordinarily verbalized in this way, this is what hatha yoga teachers want you to do. It is the preferred beginning step for forward bending, whether standing or sitting. Only after this subtle maneuver is accomplished, should you bend forward at the hips and then the spine. As you bend forward at the latter sites, the sacroiliac joints will readjust themselves, moving to a more neutral position between nutation and counternutation.

The Downward-Facing Dog works especially well for evaluating and sensing sacroiliac movements in advanced students, because experts have enough hip flexibility to settle into the posture with an arched-forward back. From this position, they can go back and forth between counternutation (pulling the ischia together, tightening the abdominal muscles and pressing the promontory of the sacrum to the rear in relation to the ilia) and nutation (sharply pulling the lumbar lordosis and sacral promontory forward with the psoas muscles, relaxing the abdominal muscles and allowing the ischia to be drawn apart). It is useful for the advanced student to keep the thighs moderately abducted for the posture, because as described earlier, an observer can monitor the movements of the upper thighs by feel: they shift medially during counternutation and laterally during nutation. Keep in mind, however, that the Downward-Facing Dog does not work well for those who are not flexible because the hoop-shaped dog posture favors pulling the ilia laterally and forward, thus creating a priority for counternutation. The remedy is simple: place the hands on a chair or table so there is plenty of leeway to keep a prominent lumbar lordosis.

We can see good potential for nutation in many postures that contain elements of forward bending from the hips. For those who are flexible enough to keep a deep lumbar lordosis during forward bends, such postures include the superfish leg lift and the straight-backed boat. And for those who are less flexible, simple and useful postures include cat stretches with maximum lumbar lordotic curvatures, sitting on your heels or on a bench in the adamantine posture and any seated meditation posture in which you can demonstrate a deep lumbar lordosis, whether you accomplish this by virtue of excellent native hip flexibility or a supporting cushion. In the cat stretches and sitting postures, even beginners can learn to relax the abdominal muscles, pitch the lumbar region and the promontory of the sacrum forward with a selective contraction of the psoas muscles, permit the ilia to come closer together and spread the ischia. Another benefit is that these simple postures permit you to alternate full nutation with full counternutation: pushing the lumbar region maximally forward favors nutation, and pushing it maximally to the rear favors counternutation.

## Nutation in Backbends

If you have a healthy back, you can do relaxed symmetrical backbending postures to encourage nutation. These include all the gravitationally-aided backbending poses, beginning with the relaxed standing lumbar bend, in which nutation accentuates the lumbar lordosis, squeezes the promontory of the sacrum forward between the ilia and spreads the ischial tuberosities. Or try this: stand with the thighs comfortably abducted and place your hands astride the ilia with the thumbs against and directly behind the top of the sacrum. Relax and bend backward to produce maximum nutation. You may not be altogether certain of feeling the top of the sacrum moving forward in relation to the ilia as you bend backward, but as you slowly shift forward from the extremity of the backbend and move into counternutation, you'll feel a dramatic shift of the ilia as they move forward and laterally on either side of the sacrum. It almost feels like a gear shifting in the manual transmission of an automobile. Another excellent posture favoring nutation is the propped, diaphragm-restricted backbend leaning against a wall, except that here you modify the posture by aiming for a diaphragm-assisted backbend. You do this by bending the knees, working your hands somewhat further down the wall and relaxing the abdomen to permit the diaphragm to accentuate the bend. This creates full nutation by squeezing the promontory of the sacrum forward in relation to the ilia. Next, try the variation of the Upward-Facing Dog in which the feet and toes are extended (the tops of the feet facing down) and the knees are left on the floor. In this posture gravity does the work of dropping the pelvis, with the promontory of the sacrum leading the way and creating nutation. If you move slowly, you can also get the same feeling with the toes flexed, resting on the balls of the feet, knees and hands. Next, try lying supine with an 8.5 inch playground ball under the lumbar region. If you can relax the abdominal muscles and allow gravity to lower the upper back and pelvis toward the floor, this posture will encourage nutation; otherwise you will protect your back with an attitude of counternutation (resistant abdominal and iliacus muscles, straighter body, squeezed-together hips and spread-apart ilia).

Finally, for those who are flexible enough, push up into the wheel posture from a supine position and allow nutation to take place as a priority, with the promontory of the sacrum squeezed forward and the ischia pulled apart. The abdomen and hip flexors, especially the iliacus muscles, must be relaxed, for only under those circumstances will full nutation complement maximum spinal and hip extension. The preference for counternutation, or even sacroiliac joints that are frozen in that attitude, is a common impediment to pushing up into the wheel for many students.

[Applied anatomy: The most advanced students, such as dancers and gymnasts who are extraordinarily flexible, may be able to do this posture one better—keeping the sacroiliac joints in an attitude of partial counternutation. The most flexible students, in fact, may feel this is desirable for protecting themselves, given that full nutation may take place too readily for their comfort. We can see a continuum of possibilities for the wheel posture: inflexible beginning students who show little or no sacroiliac movement; intermediate students who can come partially into the wheel by pushing to their limits of nutation; advanced students with excellent sacroiliac mobility who feel comfortable in the posture with full nutation; and last, those who have more sacroiliac flexibility for nutation than they feel comfortable using.]

## Counternutation in Various Postures

Nutation is natural in Upward-Facing Dog, in which you support the posture between the knees and the hands, but counternutation is more natural when the Upward-Facing Dog is supported between the feet and the hands. For the latter, squeeze the hips together while keeping the toes either flexed or extended. The main object here is to engage the abdominal, gluteal and deep back muscles strongly enough to initiate coming into the posture with a relatively straight body and the fullest possible counternutation. You can feel it: the ilia are pulled forward in relation to the sacrum by the iliacus muscles, and that movement is supported by squeezing the hips together along with the ischia. Once this posture is established, lower the pelvis carefully so as not to release the counternutation. The abdominal muscles (along with the respiratory and pelvic diaphragms) will act synergistically with the iliacus muscles to support counternutation: they will resist lowering of the pelvis eccentrically but powerfully. Because in combination they maintain a high intra-abdominal pressure throughout the breathing cycle, they will also assist in keeping the lumbar spine straight and keeping the promontory of the sacrum well to the rear in relation to the ilia. Again, you can feel all of these tendencies if you have a clear concept of the anatomy. The most common postures that support counternutation are standing and sitting forward bends from the waist. All you have to do is flex the spine forward (as opposed to flexing the hips), and this will encourage counternutation. Health-club crunch exercises, the fire exercise, yoga sit-ups, the round-bottom boat, the phase of standard cat stretches that push the lower back toward the ceiling with the abdominal muscles, a relaxed and externally supported standing forward bend for beginners and the beginner's forward bend with the fists in the armpits all foster counternutation—keeping the ischia together, the ilia apart and the promontory of the sacrum to the rear. And these postures are all safe and easy. The other supremely important standing postures that support counternutation were mentioned earlier: standing whole-body backbends (as contrasted to lumbar backbends) in which the hips and ischia are squeezed together and the main priority is keeping the promontory of the sacrum to the rear and the ilia spread apart. It's another posture for those who require maximum lumbar protection, particularly when the maximum bend is accompanied by deep empowered thoracic inhalations. In general, counternutation is preferred by those who are uncertain of themselves. They keep the hips squeezed together, the pelvis tucked under in a posterior pelvic tilt and maintain tense abdominal muscles, all of which are classic postural adjustments for everyone who has a stiff back. If this describes you, don't fight the reality; go with it. This is the work you need to do. After a year or so of conditioning, you may feel inclined to pursue more postures that release counternutation and favor nutation.

## Asymmetric Postures and Therapeutic Approaches

If one sacroiliac joint is more restricted than the other, you can use asymmetric postures to free up the joint on the tight side. But you need to be careful, because it is easy to make a mistake and work selectively on the wrong side. So, to be certain of your diagnosis, first go back and forth for 20–30 minutes between postures that favor extreme nutation and others that favor extreme counternutation. Then, watch and wait for 24 hours. If you have sacroiliac discomfort only on one side in the form of a vague ache in the region of the sacroiliac joint, it probably means that the sacroiliac joint on that side is more restricted than it is on the other. Do make sure, however, that you are not feeling symptoms discussed earlier in this chapter—unilateral iliolumbar ligament strain, lower back pain on one side or sciatica. As soon as you know which sacroiliac joint is more restricted, keep working mostly on symmetric postures, but think of adding some that are asymmetric. The preliminary pigeon as well as folding forward from that posture are excellent and will tend to open up the sacroiliac joint associated with the front knee. Do them 3 times, first and last for the tight side. The best and simplest asymmetric standing posture that selectively affects one sacroiliac joint is the first stage of the angle posture in which you are initiating a bend from one hip. If the right side is tight, come forward facing the right foot only to the extent that you can maintain a full lumbar lordosis and then, pull selectively and insistently with the right psoas muscle to encourage full nutation in the right sacroiliac joint. Don't come any further forward, as this is likely to release the nutation. As usual, face the right foot, then the left, then the right once more. It is best to work with simple postures that can be analyzed without doubt. Asymmetric standing postures such as triangles, side bends and lunges, as well as asymmetric sitting postures and twists, are all so complex that it is better to work with them in each direction equally. Unless you are certain of what you are doing, you might end up favoring the wrong side.

## Hip Flexibility

Good hip flexibility is the most important requirement for at least half the postures in hatha yoga—sitting and standing forward bends, lunges, triangles, sitting spinal twists, many variations of the inverted postures and meditative sitting postures. The problem with talking about hip flexibility is that most people do not ordinarily trouble themselves to define it precisely. If students can't bend forward in the posterior stretch because of tight hamstrings, or if they cannot abduct their thighs very far because of tight adductors, or if they cannot extend their hips because of tight hip flexors or if their sacroiliac joints are frozen, is it appropriate for hatha teachers to term these problems of hip flexibility?

They usually do. But in one sense poor hip flexibility is the result, not the cause of these situations, just as hip inflexibility can be the result of excess weight in the abdomen in those who are obese.

## Balance, Stability and Mobility in the Hip Joint

Many of us sit for a living—or for far too many hours when we get home from work each night—and our hips are subject to a lot of imbalanced forces. Sitting leads to shortened hip flexors (including the psoas, iliacus, and rectus femoris) and weak hip extensors (especially the gluteus maximus), which prompts the hamstrings to work harder. The combination of all of this leads to a common set of muscle imbalances that can produce, among other things, abnormal pressures within the hip joint itself and that dreaded tightness.

Stretching the muscles that surround your hip can help to maintain healthy mobility of the joints, to improve circulation of the synovial fluid (which reduces friction in the joint cartilage during movement) and to counteract some of the imbalances created by our chronically sedentary lives. However, while maintaining range of motion in your hips is very important, it's not all about flexibility. Based on firsthand experience, both from my perspective as a doctor who treats patients with hip-joint pain and as someone with occasional hip pain myself, I'm confident stating that balancing flexibility with strength in the muscles around the hip joint is the key to mobility and stability.

To better understand, let's look at what determines mobility and stability in your hip joints. First, there is the joint shape: a ball fitted into a socket. Surrounding the bone are a capsule and tough ligaments (which connect bone to bone at the joints). Finally, there are the "dynamic" stabilizers of the joint—your muscles. Bones do not change shape, and in general, the ligaments do not stretch very much. So, if you can't change your bone shape and your ligaments and cartilage are fixed in shape and length, what can you adjust so that you can more easily get into hip-opening poses? The answer is— your muscles and tendons.

### Identify Your Own Hip Joint Imbalances

To activate the muscles in your hips—and learn where your weaknesses and imbalances are so you can ultimately find more openness—try this exercise: Come into Baddha Konasana (Bound Angle Pose). Your knees should be flexed, while your hips will be abducted and externally rotated. Now, squeeze your calves against your thighs and notice that your hamstrings contract. Next, squeeze the outsides of your hips and buttocks to draw your knees down, then notice that you'll go deeper into the pose. This exercise engages many of the muscles that create the form of the pose—including the tensor fascia latae, gluteus medius and hamstrings—and you will likely experience more "open" hips in the pose as a result.

Now, do this exercise again and notice if there is a difference between your muscles on each side. Does your right knee melt toward the floor more easily than your left? Do your left hamstrings seem weaker? On the side that feels less strong, engage your muscles a little more strongly than on your other side (while still keeping your stronger side active) to find more balance. You can apply this same observation to your hips: Are the gluteals on one side stronger than the other? If so, practice engaging the weaker glute, without letting the stronger one go slack.

## The Emotional Effects of Hip Openers

The beauty of finding more balance and openness in the hips is that not only will it lead you into your fullest expression of hip-opening poses, it will also help on an emotional level. That's because stress causes our bodies to contract and curl inward—a natural action to protect the vital organs. But hip openers counter this energetic closing, which means there is a good chance they will affect your mental state and perception of well-being for the better.

### Get Your Hips to the Perfect Props

Feel ease and increased flexibility in your hips with 3 propped hip-opening poses.

When you get up after a long stint in your desk chair or when you sit down to meditate, do your hips talk to you, telling you their tales of tight, achy woe? For most people, they do. Even if you did the Pigeon Pose yesterday, that bittersweet stretch of the outer hip and buttocks never seems to last long enough. Put in just a little time every day, though, and your hips will thank you. You'll feel more at ease in your body and your meditation practice will feel less like a chore.

The hips are constantly on the job. They're densely packed with strong muscles and tendons that keep the joints stable, but they are also mobile enough to move you around from place to place. It takes awareness and attention to strike this sweet balance between ease of movement and stability. In addition, sitting in a chair and bearing weight on your pelvis all day limits circulation, and when you don't regularly put your hips through their full range of motion, they get tight. It's essential to do more than just the occasional Pigeon to keep your hips open and agile. Here, we present 3 creative—dare we say fun?—ways to incorporate more hip-opening poses in your daily routine.

### Action Plan

The soft tissue around the pelvis is complex and multilayered. To access and stretch this intricate web of hip muscles and deep rotators, it's helpful to incorporate several poses into your regular routine. In this practice, you will focus on creating flexibility in 2 gluteal muscles (gluteus maximus and gluteus medius) and a group of 6 external rotators (piriformis, quadratus femoris, obturator internus, obturator externus, gemellus superior and gemellus inferior).

### The End Game

Your hips are the central hub of movement in your body. When they're tight, it's like wearing a pair of pants that are a size too small—the reduced range of motion in your hips, hamstrings and spine creates discomfort. Opening this region increases the efficiency of circulation to your lower extremities, provides better range of motion and helps you feel more at ease during meditation and in seated postures.

## *Before You Begin*

Since repetition is the most essential aspect of keeping the hip area flexible, these 3 postures are designed to fit easily into a daily routine. You can add them to any phase of your practice. Placing them early in a sequence will prepare you for standing poses, twists and forward bends. But if you prefer to warm up first, you can finish your practice with the poses and settle into them deeply. These 3 poses can also make up your entire practice. Don't underestimate the value of simply taking 10 minutes a day, either in the morning or in the evening, to drop into these poses.

## *1. Pigeon Pose, Variation*

**How to do:** Place a bolster along the right side of your mat and have 2 blocks nearby. Come into the pose by situating your right sitting bone, outer thigh, and knee on the bolster. Align your front shin so that it is parallel to the front of your mat. To focus the action more intensely in your hip rotators (and to minimize the possibility of overstretching your front ankle), be sure to flex your front foot. Slide your left leg toward the back edge of your mat, leveling your hips and placing your hands on blocks set shoulder-width apart in front of you.

Before deepening the pose, you may need to troubleshoot 2 areas. First, if your front ankle is uncomfortable or if you feel too much weight on your shin, place a rolled mat under your outer shin, just above your ankle. This should relieve pressure on your foot and ankle. Second, if your knee is uncomfortable or if you're unable to place your front shin parallel to the front of your mat, pull your front heel toward your hips.

Once you settle into the pose, observe the location and intensity of the sensations in your right hip and buttock. If possible, bring your forearms to the blocks and settle the weight of your pelvis more deeply into the bolster. Root down through your arms and lengthen your spine forward while you gently draw back through your right groin and sitting bone. Complement these actions by slightly twisting your trunk to the right. This movement will create a more intense stretch in the deep layers of your outer hip. Stay for 1–2 minutes, breathing smoothly, before changing sides.

**Why This Works:** This propping typically makes it easier to bring the front shin parallel to the front edge of your mat, which will encourage your thighbone to externally rotate more. Setting up this way will also give you more access to some of the deeper external rotators of your hip. Since everybody is unique, it's normal for you to feel the stretch in a slightly different place than your neighbor.

## *2. Ankle-to-Knee on Chair*

**How to do:** You will take 3 versions of this pose to emphasize slightly different muscles in the outer hips and buttocks. Notice which version brings up the greatest resistance, and be willing to repeat that version more consistently in your daily practice.

To prepare, sit on the front edge of the chair with your knees hip-width apart and your feet directly under your knees. Place your right ankle on top of your left knee and flex your foot to maintain the alignment of your ankle and knee.

To enter the first phase of the posture, place your hands behind you on the chair seat or press them against the rungs of the chair back. Root down through your sitting bones, lengthen your spine and tilt your pelvis forward. As you hinge forward, imagine that you are going to extend your heart beyond your front shin. Glance at your front ankle and make sure that you are maintaining your flexed foot, which should prevent your ankle from rolling out. Relax your jaw, eyes and abdomen as you settle into the opening. Take 5 to 6 smooth breaths before entering the second phase of the pose.

Continuing to drop more deeply into the feeling of your body and breath, take your left hand and press it against the bottom of your right foot for the second phase of the posture. As your left hand presses your right foot, return the favor: Use your right foot to press into your hand. There will be no actual movement of the hand or foot, but the reciprocal actions will intensify the stretch and slightly shift its location. Reground your sitting bones, lift your chest by 1–2 inches and elongate your torso. Notice the sensations—they're probably pretty hard to miss at this point—and deepen your breath for 5 to 6 more rounds.

For the last phase of the pose, wrap your left arm underneath your right shin and hold on to your right kneecap with your left hand. Place your right hand on your right thigh near your hip crease. Lift your torso slightly, gently twist toward your right leg and press your hand against your thigh to add leverage to your rotation. Adding this twist will create an even deeper external rotation in your right hip. Intensify the opening by gently pulling your right hip crease with your right hand; turning your torso deeper into the twist and leaning your upper body slightly back. Notice how this final version complements the previous versions by slightly altering the focus of the stretch. Drop into your breaths for 5 to 6 rounds before releasing the posture and switching sides.

**Why This Works:** A chair provides you with excellent stability and leverage for working deeply into your glutes and hip rotators, especially if you find it difficult to sit on the floor. This is also a great alternative if hip-opening poses typically cause discomfort in your knees.

## 3. Ankle-to-Knee at Wall

**How to do:** Finding the appropriate distance from the wall will likely require a little trial and error. If you are too close to it, your hips will begin to lift off the floor; if you're too far from it, you won't receive a sufficient enough stretch. Keep this in mind and adjust your body accordingly as you nestle into the pose.

To prepare, cozy up to a wall. Lie on your back, bend your knees and place your feet on the wall. You'll find the greatest amount of comfort if you place your feet so that your shins are perpendicular to the wall. Meanwhile, your sitting bones should be as close the wall as you can get them.

Press your feet into the wall, lift your hips and place your right ankle on your left knee. You're about to initiate the process of sliding away from the wall until you hit your sweet spot. Once you have your right ankle on top of your knee, gradually inch away from the wall until your lower back and sacrum touch the floor. If you go too far too quickly, you will lose the stretch in your hip, so be sure to move slowly and deliberately. Once the backs of your hips touch the floor, root down firmly with your sacrum and tilt the front rim of your pelvis forward. You might not feel any discernible movement in your hips, but the action will intensify the stretch. Check your left leg to make sure that your shin is perpendicular to the wall. Flex your right foot and see that your ankle is not rolling out.

Cross your arms overhead and rest your forearms on the floor (or place one hand on your abdomen and the other on your heart) as you relax the rest of your body into the floor. Direct your awareness and breathe into your right hip, encouraging the tissues to soften and release. Stay for up to 3 minutes before changing sides.

**Why This Works:** Reclining in this pose allows you to exert a minimal amount of effort while you get a nice stretch in your hips and buttocks. Since the pose does not require a significant output of energy, you can hold it for a while, accessing deeper layers of resistance while settling into your breath.

To work on activating the muscles of the hips to find more balance, try this sequence.

## Anjaneyasana (Low Lunge)

Step the left foot back into a lunge, bending the right knee directly over the right heel and bringing the left knee to the floor (you can use a folded blanket under the knee for comfort). Engage the left glutes to increase the stretch in the front of the left hip. Bend the left knee and grasp the ankle with your hand or a strap to deepen the hip stretch. Then activate the muscles by imagining that you are trying to drag the left knee forward. Hold for 5 seconds, then relax and go deeper into the stretch. Release and repeat on the other side.

## Upavistha Konasana (Wide-Angle Seated Forward Bend)

This pose stretches the hamstrings and the adductor muscles on the inner thighs. Sit on the floor with your legs in a V and activate your quadriceps to straighten the knees. Engage the outer hip muscles to widen the legs, then press your heels into the floor and attempt to drag them toward each other isometrically to contract the hamstrings and adductors. Hold for 5 seconds, relax, then repeat and go deeper into the stretch.

## Setu Bandha Sarvangasana (Bridge Pose)

This pose strengthens the outer hip and gluteal muscles. Lie on your back with your knees bent and feet hip-distance apart. Press your feet into the floor and attempt to drag them apart without movement. This trains the outer hip muscles to remain active in the pose and strengthens the muscles around the pelvis. Maintain this action as you contract the gluteus maximus to lift the pelvis up into Bridge. Hold for 5 breaths and release.

## Eka Pada Rajakapotasana (Pigeon Pose)

This pose stretches the outer hip and gluteals and relieves tension in the deep hip muscles. From Tabletop, bring your right ankle toward your left wrist and place the lower right leg on the floor parallel to the front edge of your mat. Extend your left leg straight behind you. You can stay lifted in a backbend or fold forward over the bent right leg. Feel free to place a block under the front thigh muscles of the extended back leg for support. Hold for 5–10 slow breaths and then repeat on the other side.

## *Pelvic Floor Muscles*

Having strong pelvic floor muscles gives us control over the bladder and bowel. Weakened pelvic floor muscles mean the internal organs are not fully supported and you may have difficulty controlling the release of urine, feces (poo) or flatus (wind).

Common causes of a weakened pelvic floor include childbirth, obesity and the associated straining of chronic constipation. Pelvic floor exercises are designed to improve muscle tone and prevent the need for corrective surgery.

What are pelvic floor muscles?

Pelvic floor muscles are the layer of muscles that support the pelvic organs and span the bottom of the pelvis. The pelvic organs are the bladder and bowel in men and bladder, bowel and uterus in women. The diagram below shows the pelvic organs and pelvic floor muscles in women (right) and men (left).

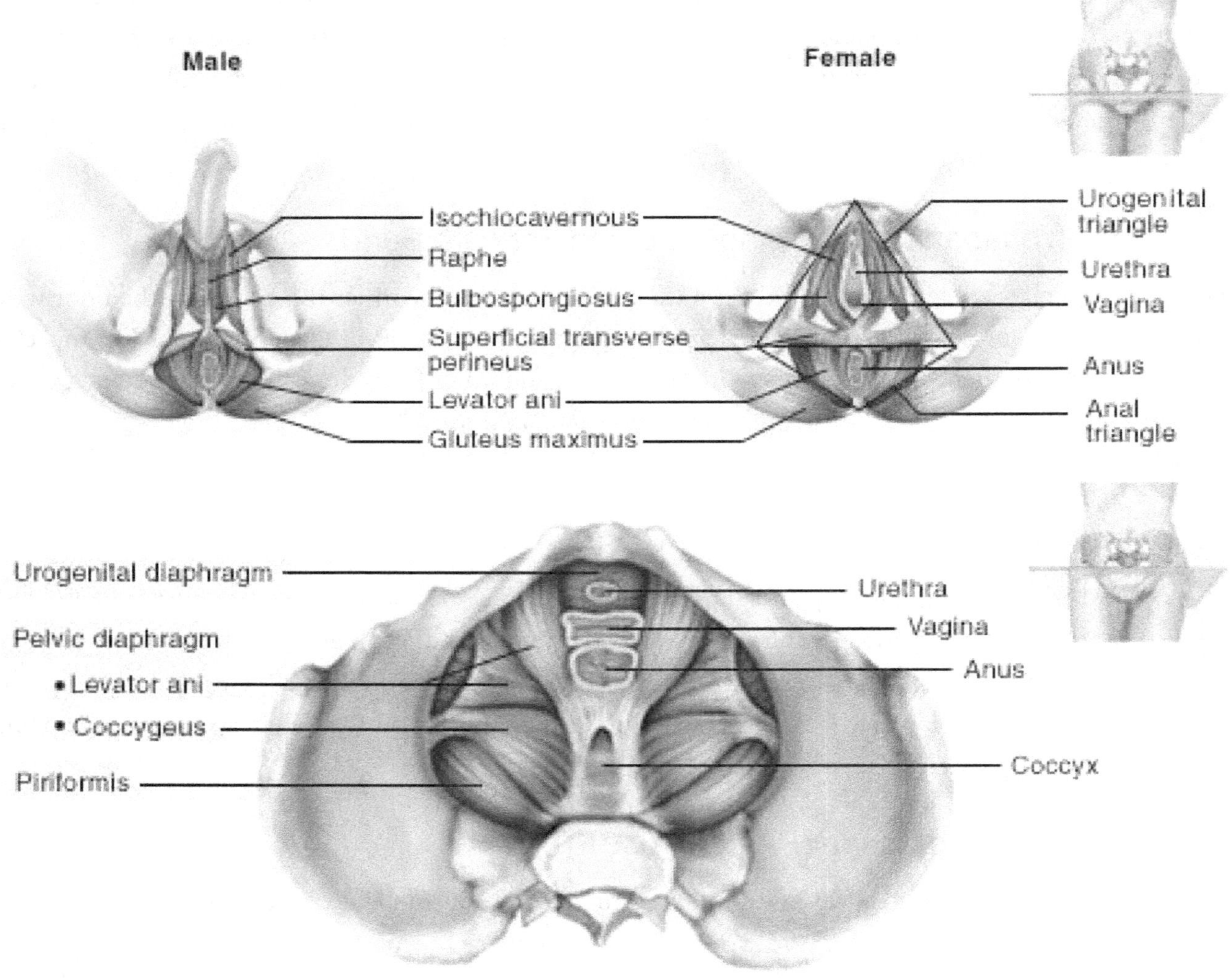


Male and female pelvic floor muscles diagram

The pelvic floor muscles stretch like a muscular trampoline from the tailbone (coccyx) to the pubic bone (front to back) and from one sitting bone to the other sitting bone (side to side). These muscles are normally firm and thick.

Imagine the pelvic floor muscles as a round mini-trampoline made of firm muscle. Just like a trampoline, the pelvic floor is able to move down and up. The bladder, uterus (for women) and bowel lie on the pelvic floor muscle layer.

The pelvic floor muscle layer has a hole for passages. There are 2 passages in men (the urethra and anus) and 3 in women (the urethra, vagina and anus). The pelvic floor muscles normally wrap quite firmly around these holes to help keep the passages shut. There is also an extra circular muscle around the anus (the anal sphincter) and around the urethra (the urethral sphincter).

Although the pelvic floor is hidden from view, it can be consciously controlled and therefore trained, much like our arm, leg or abdominal muscles.

What do pelvic floor muscles do?

Pelvic floor muscles provide support to the organs that lie on it. The sphincters give us conscious control over the bladder and bowel so that we can control the release of urine, feces (poo) and flatus (wind) and allow us to delay emptying until it is convenient. When the pelvic floor muscles are contracted, internal organs are lifted and the sphincters tighten the openings of the vagina, anus and urethra. Relaxing the pelvic floor allows passage of urine and feces.

Pelvic floor muscles are also important for sexual function in both men and women. In men, it is important for erectile function and ejaculation. In women, voluntary contractions (squeezing) of the pelvic floor contribute to sexual sensation and arousal.

The pelvic floor muscles in women also provide support for the baby during pregnancy and assist in the birthing process.

The muscles of the pelvic floor work with the abdominal and back muscles to stabilize and support the spine. So, tone in these muscles translates into stability for the sacroiliac joint and the spine too.

# The Spine

The spine is made up of 33 individual bones stacked one on top of the other. This spinal column provides the main support for your body, allowing you to stand upright, bend and twist, while protecting the spinal cord from injury. Strong muscles and bones, flexible tendons and ligaments and sensitive nerves contribute to a healthy spine. Yet, any of these structures affected by strain, injury or disease can cause pain.

## Spinal Curves

When viewed from the side, an adult spine has a natural S-shaped curve. The neck (cervical) and lower back (lumbar) regions have a slight concave curve (lordotic) and the thoracic and sacral regions have a gentle convex curve (kyphotic). The curves work like a coiled spring to absorb shock, maintain balance and allow range of motion throughout the spinal column.

# Human vertebral column

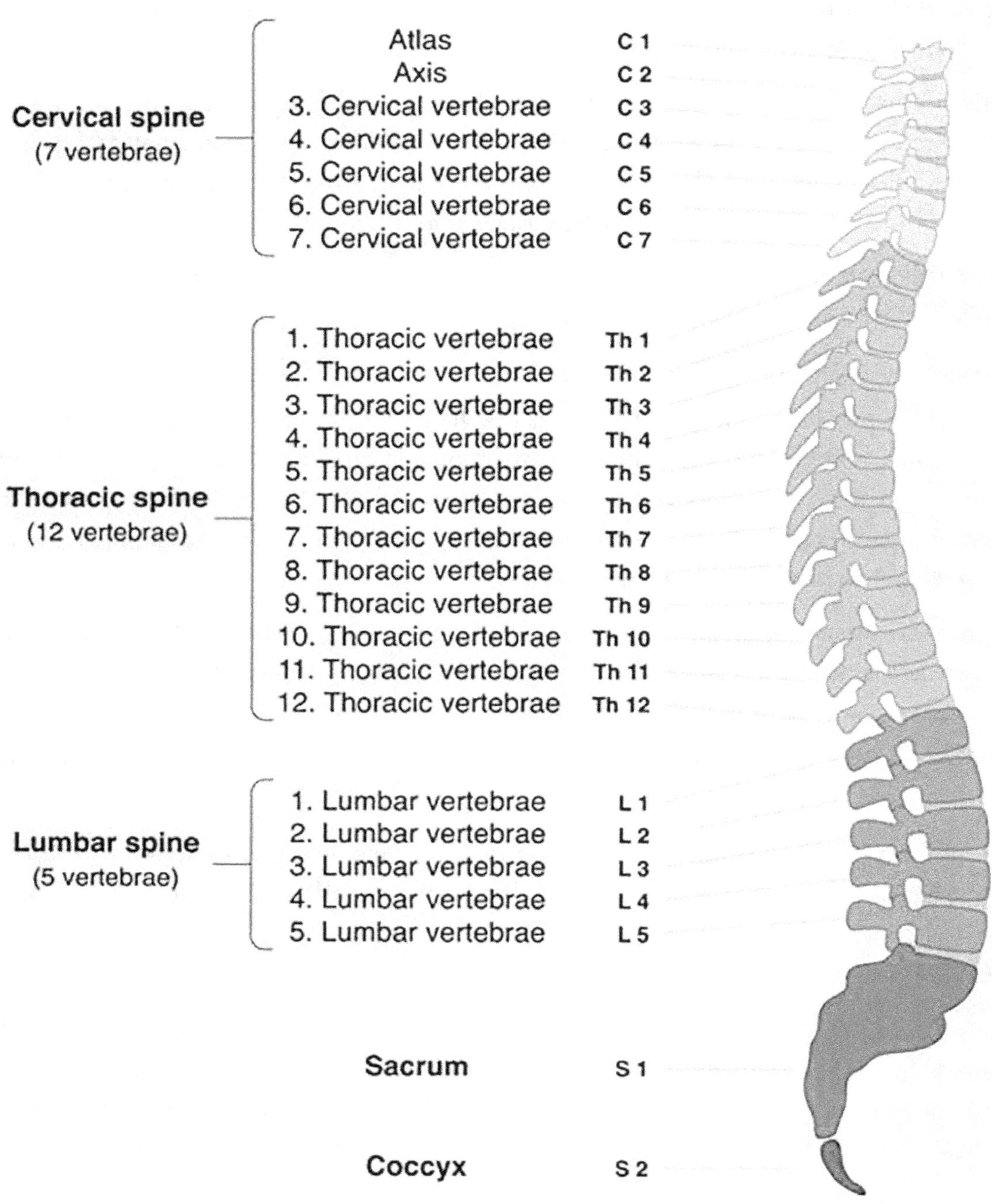



The muscles and correct posture maintain natural spinal curves. Good posture involves training your body to stand, walk, sit and lie so that the least amount of strain is placed on the spine during movement or weight-bearing activities (see Posture). Excess body weight, weak muscles, and other forces can pull at the spine's alignment.

## *Spinal Muscles*

The 2 main muscle groups that affect the spine are extensors and flexors. The extensor muscles enable us to stand up and lift objects. The extensors are attached to the back of the spine. The flexor muscles are in the front and include the abdominal muscles. These muscles enable us to flex or bend forward and are important in lifting and controlling the arch in the lower back.

# Muscles of the Back

- Erector spinae group
    - 3 columns muscle
    - extends from sacrum to ribs
    - extends vertebral column
- Semispinalis group
    - vertebrae to vertebrae
    - extends neck
- Multifidis
    - vertebrae to vertebrae
    - rotates vertebral column
- Quadratus lumborum
    - ilium to 12th rib
    - lateral flexion

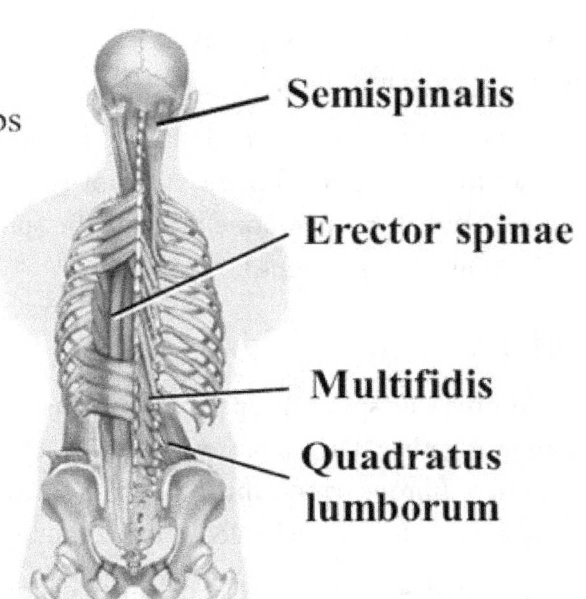


The back muscles stabilize your spine. Something as common as poor muscle tone or a large belly can pull your entire body out of alignment. Misalignment puts incredible strain on the spine.

## *Vertebrae*

Vertebrae are the 33 individual bones that interlock with each other to form the spinal column. The vertebrae are numbered and divided into regions: cervical, thoracic, lumbar, sacrum and coccyx. Only the top 24 bones are moveable; the vertebrae of the sacrum and coccyx are fused. The vertebrae in each region have unique features that help them perform their main functions.

Cervical (neck): the main function of the cervical spine is to support the weight of the head (about 10 pounds). The seven cervical vertebrae are numbered C1 to C7. The neck has the greatest range of motion because of 2 specialized vertebrae that connect to the skull. The first vertebra (C1) is the ring-shaped atlas that connects directly to the skull. This joint allows for the nodding or "yes" motion of the head. The second vertebra (C2) is the peg-shaped axis, which has a projection called the odontoid, that the atlas pivots around. This joint allows for the side-to-side or "no" motion of the head.

Thoracic (mid-back): the main function of the thoracic spine is to hold the rib cage and protect the heart and lungs. The twelve thoracic vertebrae are numbered T1 to T12. The range of motion in the thoracic spine is limited.

Lumbar (lower back): the main function of the lumbar spine is to bear the weight of the body. The 5 lumbar vertebrae are numbered L1 to L5. These vertebrae are much larger in size to absorb the stress of lifting and carrying heavy objects.

Sacrum: the main function of the sacrum is to connect the spine to the hip bones (iliac). There are 5 sacral vertebrae, which are fused together. Together with the iliac bones, they form a ring called the pelvic girdle.

Coccyx region: the 4 fused bones of the coccyx or tailbone provide attachment for the ligaments and muscles of the pelvic floor.

While vertebrae have unique regional features, every vertebra has 3 main parts: body, vertebral arch and processes for muscle attachment. A drum-shaped body is designed to bear weight and withstand compression. An arch-shaped bone protects the spinal cord. A star-shaped process is designed as an outrigger for muscle attachment.

## Intervertebral discs

Each vertebra in your spine is separated and cushioned by an intervertebral disc, keeping the bones from rubbing together. Discs are designed like a radial car tire. The outer ring, called the annulus, has crisscrossing fibrous bands, much like a tire tread. These bands attach between the bodies of each vertebra. Inside the disc is a gel-filled center called the nucleus, much like a tire tube.

Intervertebral discs are made of a gel-filled center called the nucleus and a tough fibrous outer ring called the annulus. The annulus pulls the vertebral bodies together against the resistance of the gel-filled nucleus.

Discs function like coiled springs. The crisscrossing fibers of the annulus pull the vertebral bodies together against the elastic resistance of the gel-filled nucleus. The nucleus acts like a ball-bearing when you move, allowing the vertebral bodies to roll over the incompressible gel. The gel-filled nucleus is composed mostly of fluid. This fluid is absorbed during the night as you lie down and is pushed out during the day as you move upright.

With age, our discs increasingly lose the ability to reabsorb fluid and become brittle and flatter; this is why we get shorter as we grow older. Also, diseases, such as osteoarthritis and osteoporosis, cause bone spurs (osteophytes) to grow. Injury and strain can cause discs to bulge or herniate, a condition in which the nucleus is pushed out through the annulus to compress the nerve roots, causing back pain.

## Vertebral Arch and Spinal Canal

On the back of each vertebra are bony projections that form the vertebral arch. The arch is made of 2 supporting pedicles and 2 laminas. The hollow spinal canal contains the spinal cord, fat, ligaments and blood vessels. Under each pedicle, a pair of spinal nerves exits the spinal cord and passes through the intervertebral foramen to branch out to your body.

# Vertebra and the Spinal Cord

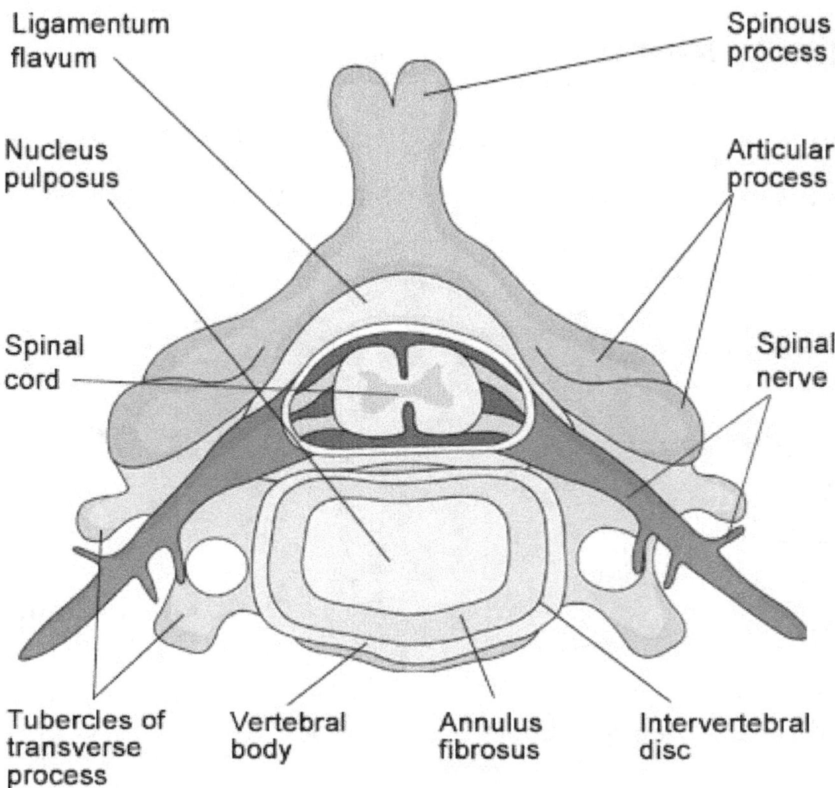


The vertebral arch forms the spinal canal through which the spinal cord runs. Seven bony processes arise from the vertebral arch to form the facet joints and processes for muscle attachment.

Surgeons often remove the lamina of the vertebral arch (laminectomy) to access and decompress the spinal cord and nerves to treat spinal stenosis, tumors or herniated discs.

Seven processes arise from the vertebral arch: the spinous process, 2 transverse processes, 2 superior facets and 2 inferior facets.

## Facet Joints

The facet joints of the spine allow back motion. Each vertebra has 4 facet joints, one pair that connects to the vertebra above (superior facets) and one pair that connects to the vertebra below (inferior facets).

The superior and inferior facets connect each vertebra together. There are four facet joints associated with each vertebra.

## Ligaments

The ligaments are strong fibrous bands that hold the vertebrae together, stabilize the spine, and protect the discs. The 3 major ligaments of the spine are the ligamentum flavum, anterior longitudinal ligament (ALL) and posterior longitudinal ligament (PLL). The ALL and PLL are continuous bands that run from the top to the bottom of the spinal column along the vertebral bodies. They prevent excessive movement of the vertebral bones.

## Vertebral Column: Ligaments

- Anterior (ventral) and posterior (dorsal) longitudinal ligaments
- Short ligaments connect adjoining vertebrae together

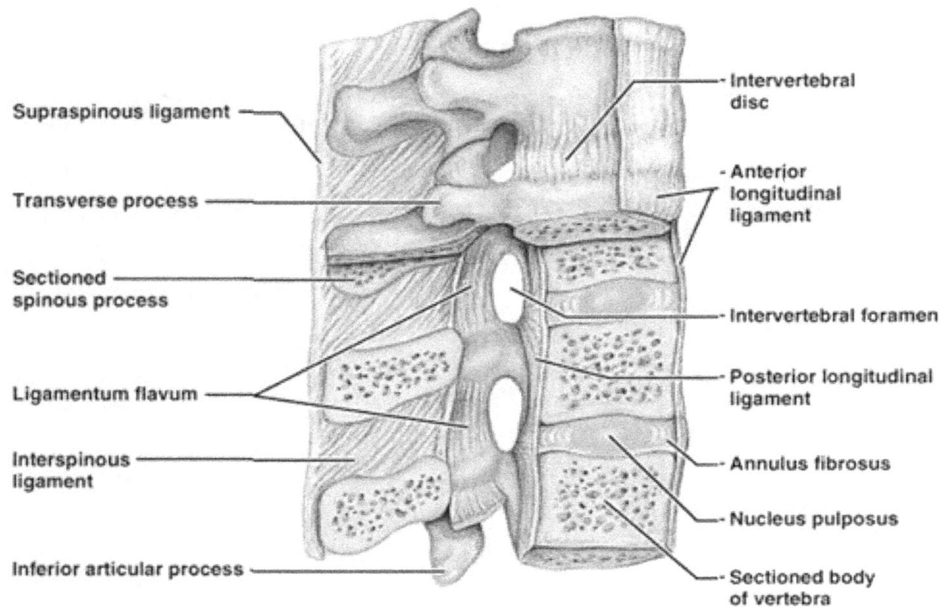


The ligamentum flavum attaches between the lamina of each vertebra. The ligamentum flavum, ALL and PLL allow the flexion and extension of the spine while keeping the vertebrae in alignment.

## Spinal Cord

The spinal cord is about 18 inches long and is as thick as your thumb. It runs within the protective spinal canal from the brainstem to the first lumbar vertebra. At the end of the spinal cord, the cord fibers separate into the cauda equina and continue down through the spinal canal to your tailbone before branching off to your legs and feet. The spinal cord serves as an information super-highway, relaying messages between the brain and the body. The brain sends motor messages to the limbs and body through the spinal cord allowing for movement. The limbs and body send sensory messages to the brain through the spinal cord about what we feel and touch. Sometimes the spinal cord can react without sending information to the brain. These special pathways, called spinal reflexes, are designed to immediately protect our body from harm.

The nerve cells that make up the spinal cord itself are called upper motor neurons. The nerves that branch off your spinal cord down your back and neck are called lower motor neurons. These nerves exit between each of your vertebrae and go to all parts of your body.

Any damage to the spinal cord can result in a loss of sensory and motor function below the level of injury. For example, an injury to the thoracic or lumbar area may cause motor and sensory loss of the legs and trunk (called paraplegia). An injury to the cervical (neck) area may cause sensory and motor loss of the arms and legs (called tetraplegia, formerly known as quadriplegia).

## Spinal Nerves

Thirty-one pairs of spinal nerves branch off the spinal cord. The spinal nerves act as "telephone lines," carrying messages back and forth between your body and spinal cord to control sensation and movement. Each spinal nerve has 2 roots. The ventral (front) root carries motor impulses from the brain and the dorsal (back) root carries sensory impulses to the brain. The ventral and dorsal roots fuse together to form a spinal nerve, which travels down the spinal canal, alongside the cord, until it reaches its exit hole—the intervertebral foramen. Once the nerve passes through the intervertebral foramen, it branches; each branch has both motor and sensory fibers. The smaller branch (called the posterior primary ramus) turns posteriorly to supply the skin and muscles at the back of the body. The larger branch (called the anterior primary ramus) turns anteriorly to supply the skin and muscles at the front of the body and forms most of the major nerves.

The ventral (motor) and dorsal (sensory) roots join to form the spinal nerve. The spinal cord is covered by 3 layers of meninges: pia, arachnoid and dura mater.

The spinal nerves are numbered according to the vertebrae above which it exits the spinal canal. The 8 cervical spinal nerves are C1 through C8, the 12 thoracic spinal nerves are T1 through T12, the 5 lumbar spinal nerves are L1 through L5 and the 5 sacral spinal nerves are S1 through S5. There is 1 coccygeal nerve.

The spinal nerves exit the spinal canal through the intervertebral foramen below each pedicle. The spinal nerves innervate specific areas and form a striped pattern across the body called dermatomes. Doctors use this pattern to diagnose the location of a spinal problem based on the area of pain or muscle weakness. For example, leg pain (sciatica) usually indicates a problem near the L4–S3 nerves.

A dermatome pattern shows which spinal nerves are responsible for sensory and motor control of specific areas of the body.

## Coverings and Spaces

The spinal cord is covered with the same 3 membranes as the brain, called meninges. The inner membrane is the pia mater, which is intimately attached to the cord. The next membrane is the arachnoid mater. The outer membrane is the tough dura mater. Between these membranes are spaces used in diagnostic and treatment procedures. The space between the pia and arachnoid mater is the wide subarachnoid space, which surrounds the spinal cord and contains cerebrospinal fluid (CSF). This space is most often accessed when performing a lumbar puncture to sample and test CSF or during a myelogram to inject contrast dye. The space between the dura mater and the bone is the epidural space. This space is most often accessed to deliver anesthetic numbing agents, commonly called an epidural, and to inject steroid medication.

## *Disorders Affecting Inter-Vertebral Discs, Herniated and Bulging Discs*

# DAMAGE TO THE SPINE

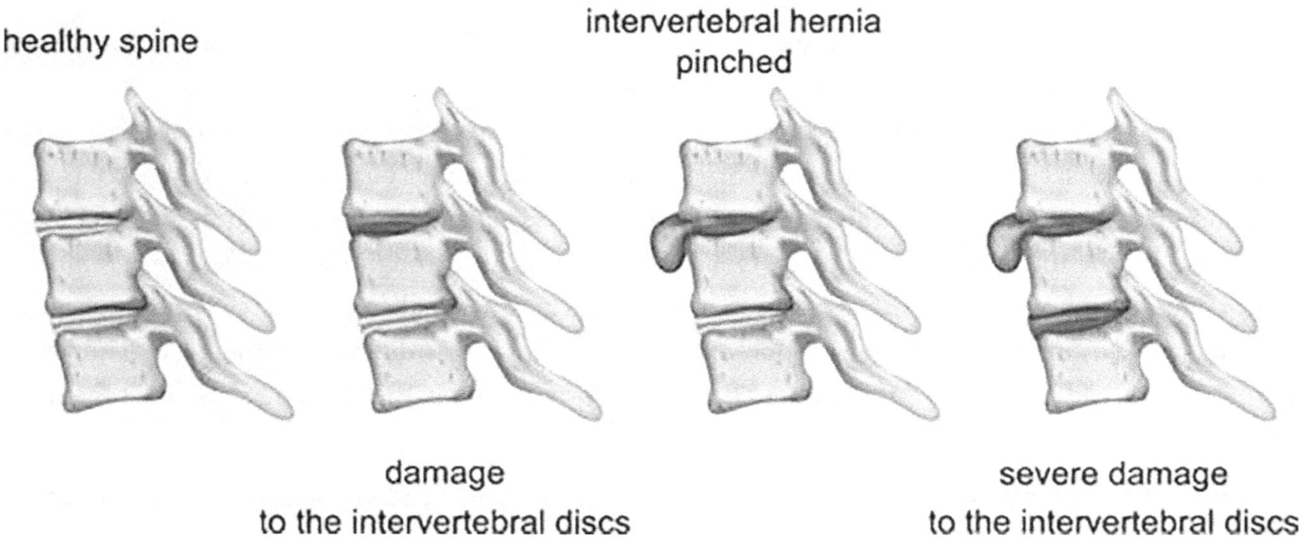


A slipped disc can mean a ruptured disc or herniated disc (pronounced "her-kneeate-ed"). Contrary to the name "slipped disc," discs do not slip. Each inter-vertebral disc is sandwiched between 2 vertebrae supported by a system of ligaments that help hold the spinal package together.

Disc disorders are contained or non-contained. A bulging disc is an example of a contained disc disorder. It has not yet broken open—the nucleus pulposus remains contained within the annulus fibrosus. It could be compared to a volcano prior to eruption and may be a precursor to herniation. The disc may protrude into the spinal canal without breaking open. The gel-like interior (nucleus pulposus) does not leak out. Instead, the disc remains intact except a small bubble pops out attached to the disc. A non-contained disc is one that has either partially or completely broken open—a herniated or ruptured disc. For example, imagine a tube (annulus fibrosus) of toothpaste (nucleus pulposus) placed under pressure. The pressure causes the toothpaste within the tube to move wherever it can. If any part of the tube is weak toothpaste may leak out. When a disc herniates, the contents may spread out to the spinal cord and nerves. The disc material has little space to go—the area occupied by the spinal canal and nerve roots.

Continuing the metaphor of the leaky toothpaste tube, the disc's gel-like nucleus contains a chemical that irritates the nerves, causing them to swell. After the chemical agent has done its job, the remnants of the chemical remain and continue to press on the irritated and swollen nerves. To complicate matters, sometimes fragments from the annulus (tire-like outer disc wall) break away from the parent disc and drift into the spinal canal. These fragments may travel in the spinal canal, and depending on the type of injury and the condition of the discs, more than one disc may herniate, rupture or bulge. Sometimes injury causes a combination of disc disorders. There are five stages of disc herniation.

## The Five Stages of Disc Herniation

Stage I: Slight movement of the gel within the envelope with no peripheral neurological signs and symptoms—often pain free. These symptoms include: muscle atrophy, tingling, numbness, loss of control and sensitivity to heat and cold.

Stage II: Larger movement of the nuclear gel but still contained within the annular ring; mild back pain.

Stage III: Mild to moderate protrusion of the nuclear material; back and leg pain is present without true positive neurological signs.

Stage IV: Disc bulges, impinging on the nerve root with positive neurological signs and back pain.

Stage V: A disc extrusion or sequestration where the nuclear material has left the annular ring; back pain actually diminishes while neurological signs and symptoms extend more peripherally and intensify.

The disc, especially in the lumbar spine, often protrudes posteriorly and laterally and can be a result of flattening the lumbar curve with an overstretched posterior longitudinal ligament.

A constant pain in the lower back and uncontrollable weakness in the legs or feet is a common symptom for people who suffer from a herniated disc. Although the symptoms can be different, the cause is often the same – a disc in the spine has herniated and is exerting pressure on a nerve root.

Most lumbar herniation is the result of years of pressure exerted on the lower spine, the area of the back that gets the most usage. Gravity, weight, and bad posture over a period of time tend to take their toll and we as humans also tend to rely more on the lower back than the rest of the spine for strength activities such as lifting heavy objects and reaching for things. Over time, the back simply gets tired and "gives out" in an attempt to inform the body that it is tired.

The following image depicts injuries at different sites of the spinal vertebrae and resulting diseases.

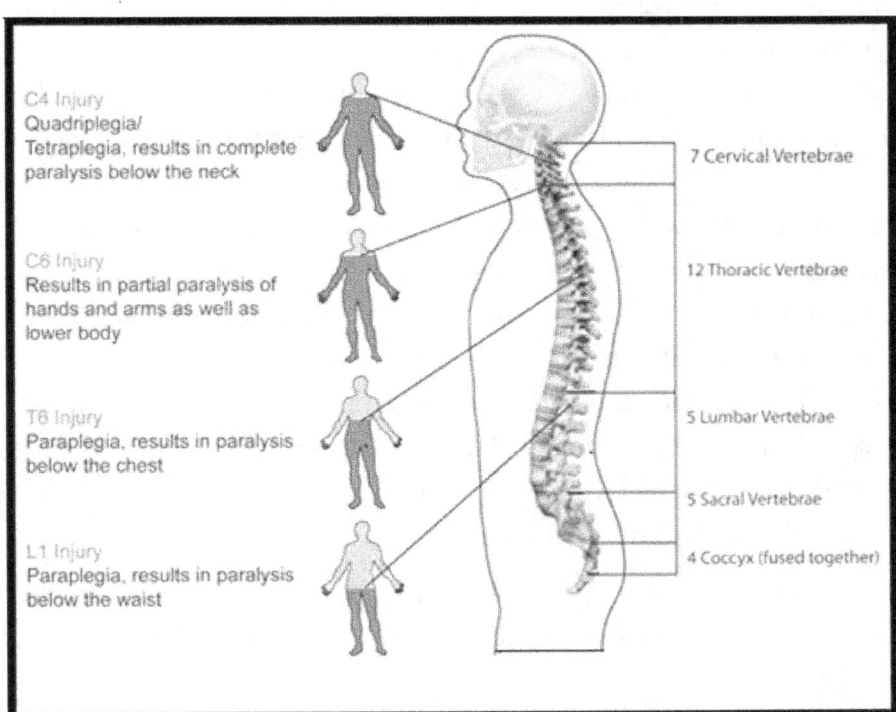

According to Ayurveda, all joint/disc injuries are a *vata* imbalance. ***Yoga Sutras,* Chapter II, V. 47 states:** "Yoga Pose is mastered by relaxation of effort, lessening the tendency for restless breathing, and promoting an identification of oneself as living within the infinite breath of life." As a result of this *vata* imbalance, the breath or prana is also affected and should, therefore, be considered as a way to heal through Yoga Therapy.

Standing poses would be very important here. Other poses would be poses that decompress the spine (work in neutral and elongated spine positions). The first focus would be "stability before mobility"—working on stabilizing the pelvis and spine and then adding dynamic movement later. Another method would be to work on the abdominal muscles because they are usually lethargic and/or weak with this population. Additionally, with degenerative disc disease of the lumbar spine, the sacrum usually becomes rigid as it attempts to support the entire spine. Another approach towards this population would be to create as much intervertebral space as possible in the lumbar spine, to allow the sacrum to be free to drop downward and thereby also releasing itself from L5. Additionally, a "whole picture" view and approach would be towards decompression of the entire spine and not just the area that is affected.

Yoga poses incorporating both static and dynamic movements and balancing poses are also very important for this population.

## Contraindications—Modify or Eliminate

Exercises that compress the spine should be avoided. Therefore, abdominal crunches and full sit ups are contraindicated. Poses involving excessive spinal flexion, especially lumbar flexion, should be avoided, as they can do further damage to already damaged discs. Forward bends should generally be avoided, unless they can be taught with a neutral spine. Additionally, when doing a forward bend such as Pashimottanasa, the first instruction should be to root the sit bones to the floor and lengthen the spine on an inhale. This elongation and lengthening should be kept while moving into the pose and the client should go only as far as needed. If the thoracic spine begins to round, the client would need to move back to where the entire spine stays in a neutral position and would only go forward a few inches. Blanket(s) should also be placed under the client's buttocks to facilitate neutral spine and to release the hip flexors. Poses like Uttanasana, Ardha Parsvottonasa and Prasarita Padottanasana can be taught with hands placed on the wall, and the client would only come as far as the torso is parallel to the floor. Apanasana, a normally contraindicated pose, can be taught one leg at a time, keeping the spine in neutral as a modification. In addition, a note here would be to make sure each knee stays in line with the hip while doing the asana. With prone back-bending poses it is important to place a blanket under the hips/pelvis to ease any pressure on the lumbar spine. The general principle in all yoga poses is the elongation of the spine (back body). A cue to elongate the front and side bodies will help here as well. Twisting poses should be approached with extreme caution and the emphasis with twists should be on elongating the spine and lifting from the ribcage.

The yoga practice needs to be both slow and mindful, to increase awareness of both the inner and outer body, as well as the breath. A vigorous vinyasa practice would be contraindicated for this population.

This population would also need to be re-educated on proper alignment principles, functional movement and body mechanics which would then positively affect their lifestyle and activities in daily living. In the end, this will also contribute to setting them free from pain.

## Scoliosis

Of all the postural changes that one might have to deal with, scoliosis is perhaps the most challenging. The father of modern medicine, Hippocrates,applied the term 'skoliosis' (crooked) to any curvature of the spine and developed methods to treat it.

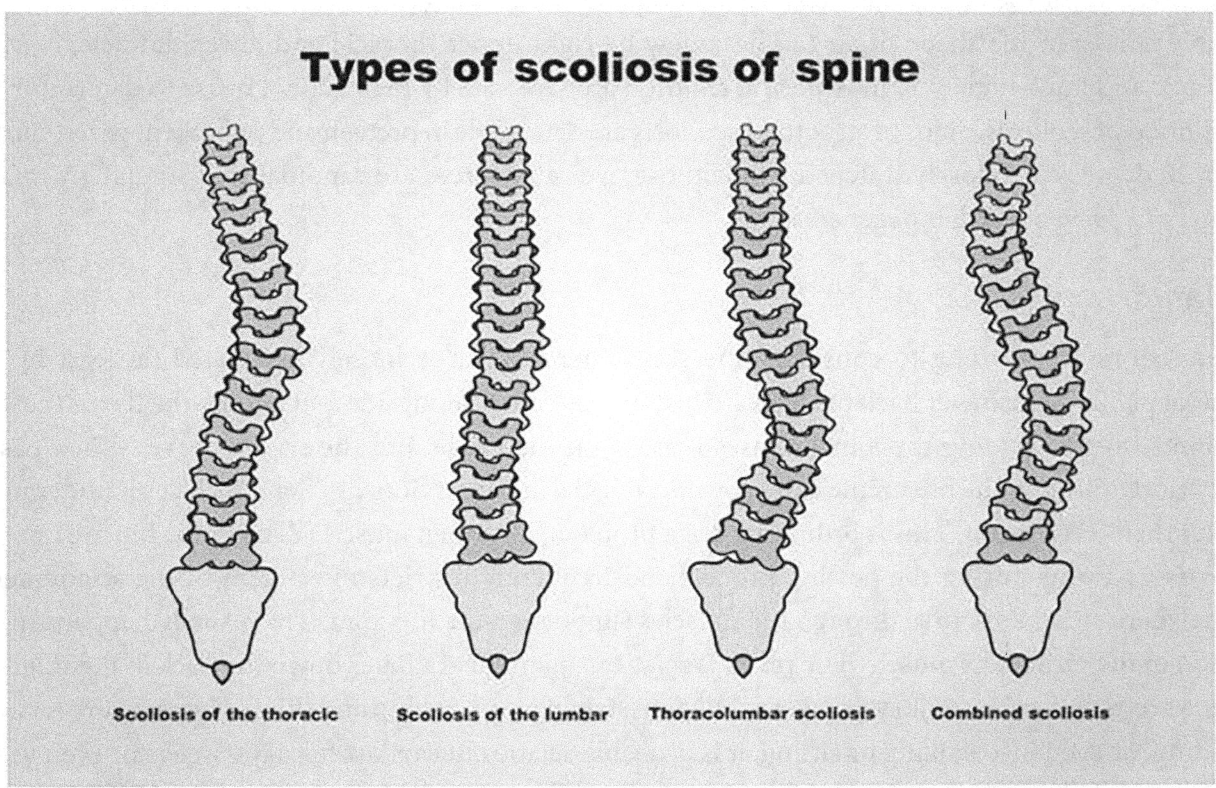



Scoliosis is a complicated deformity characterized by lateral curvature and vertebral rotation. As the disease progresses, the vertebrae and spinous processes in the area of the major curve rotate toward the concavity of the curve. The disc spaces become narrower on the concave side of the curve and wider on the convex side.

Forms of spinal deformity can be broadly classified into structural and nonstructural types. In nonstructural scoliosis, the curve is flexible and corrects on side bending toward the convex side; in structural scoliosis, the curve fails to correct on side bending.

Nonstructural scoliosis is sometimes developed as a result of a specific activity done for a long period of time. This is also called functional scoliosis. Any one-sided activity can produce this type of curvature. Examples are playing golf, bowling, tennis, racket ball, or carrying a heavy weight on just one side. This often occurs in mothers carrying their infants on the same hip, or from being a waitress and carrying a heavy tray on the same shoulder. In this type, the body's muscular and skeletal structures have been temporarily distorted to accommodate the requirements of the functional task at hand. There are usually marked differences, not only in posture (one shoulder or hip being higher), but also changes in strength and stamina from one side of the body to the other. I have seen clients with this type of curvature make dramatic changes in a relatively short period of time. When the activity causing the curvature was habitual for less than a year, the body can resume its original shape within 2–4 months of personally mentored Structural Yoga Therapy.

There are 4 varieties of curvatures. The right thoracic curve is the most common. A second is a thoracolumbar curve, characterized by a long major C curve to the right, through both the lower and upper regions of the back, in which there is only one long change of direction. The other 2 types are double curves in the shape of an S. These may be right upper thoracic and lower thoracic, or right thoracic and lumbar curves. In America, children are screened by their school nurse to determine the likelihood of scoliosis. Signs of structural scoliosis are detectable in preteen and pubescent years. Curves over 30 degrees are closely watched, while those over 45 degrees are candidates for metal bracing or surgery to prevent further degeneration.

## Sciatica

There is one more thing to consider—the sciatic nerve—that is loosely associated (at least by the general public) with lower back problems. Most nerves course alongside and among the flexor muscles of joints, so that folding the joint releases tension on the nerve. But the sciatic nerve, which passes posteriorly through the hip on the extensor side, is a glaring exception: hip flexion places it under more rather than less tension. This is ordinarily not a problem, but when muscles deep in the hip are injured, scar tissue forms during the healing process and frequently restricts movement of the sciatic nerve somewhere along its course through the muscles supporting the hip joint. This usually happens in the region of the piriformis muscle. The result is sciatica—pain that radiates down the back of the thigh. If, after a seemingly minor injury, you get a dull persistent pain in one hip and thigh when you are forward bending, or even just walking or sitting, it is probably sciatica. It can last for days, weeks or even years, but assuming the source of the problem is in the hips, it can usually be treated successfully by manual medicine and bodywork, often in combination with a program of stretching.

## Chapter 2

# THE FUNDAMENTALS OF YOGA PRACTICE: BREATH, BANDHA, DRISHTI AND VINYASA

## The Yogic Approach to Asana Practice

In *Yoga Sutra* II. 46, 47 and 48, Patanjali quotes on asana. The simplicity is profound.

"Posture is steadiness and ease."

"True posture is then when effort ceases and meditation on infinity occurs."

"In asana there is no assault from the pair of opposites."

The Ashtanga Vinyasa yoga practice is a movement meditation. The goal is that every breath taken becomes a conscious one. The sequence, the flow, holding of the bandhas, drishti and listening to the sound of the Ujjayi Pranayama are all techniques designed to withdraw the senses. Now let's analyze them in anatomical perspective.

## Breath

As quoted by Sri K. Pattabhi Jois, in his book, *Yogamala*: "The most visible aspect of Ashtanga yoga system is the different yoga asanas (postures). More important is the visible content, which consists of three fundamental techniques. These techniques bind the postures together on a string so that they become a yoga mala or garland."

For the beginner, it is essential to learn these 3 fundamental techniques. Once they are mastered, the practice will happen almost effortlessly. Without them, the practice can become hard work. The 3 techniques are Ujjayi Pranayama, Mula Bandha and Uddyana Abandha.

An important aspect of Classical Yoga is the strengthening and cultivation of the life-force energy called prana. While prana is not the breath, it is most readily discovered through the discipline of the respiratory function. This, together with the heightened sensitivity that is the hallmark of yoga training, reveals the hidden secret of the breath as prana. The word prana literally means "primary or vital air." Its prefix, "pra," means forward, toward, or prior. The suffix, "na," means to breathe or to energize. For the yogi, the vital force is in the body and it surrounds us and interpenetrates all objects. Prana can be gotten from external objects, but this type is short-lived. The yogi seeks to refine his own breath into more prana, not unlike the alchemists who sought to transform base metals into gold. Yoga is indeed alchemy; the self becomes the Self.

The practices of working with the breath to strengthen and extend respiration are the preliminary methods of yoga breathing culminating in pranayama. These exercises begin with simple breathing methods such as those a respiratory therapist might use for the alleviation of symptoms of shortness of breath or to develop a greater vital capacity in the lungs. These are quite powerful practices, given that most people breathe with as little as 25 percent of their respiratory capacity. Just increasing respiratory efficiency can provide tremendous relief to vital organs that have been starved of oxygen and pervaded with the waste gas, carbon dioxide. It's no wonder that just learning how to take deeper, fuller breaths efficiently and on a regular basis can have an uplifting effect on all physiological systems.

The practice of asanas with a full breathing technique is central to the process of Classical Yoga. This is one of the hallmarks that distinguish Classical Yoga from regular physical fitness or gymnastic exercise.

In Classical Yoga, the poses are practiced in 2 ways: using rhythmic breathing to come into and out of poses practiced in a continuous flowing sequence called vinyasa or practicing poses separately in a logical sequence, statically held, in a stable comfortable manner. According to Patanjali, the poses are perfected by a sequence of steps through which awareness of the life-force is cultivated. To find this inner pose, which creates a stable, comfortable outer posture, smooth full breathing must be developed. The breath is intimately connected to the mind. It is said, "If the breath is agitated, so is the mind." Therefore, to quiet the mind to direct its attention, we first learn to regulate the breath.

## How to Breathe

To begin the process of breath awareness, lie down on the floor in the Savasana (Corpse Pose), relax and observe the motion of your breath. Now rest your hands at your sides, separate the legs enough to relax your lower back. Observe your natural breath pattern. Let your mind begin to notice the air as it enters your nostrils. Watch where it expands as you inhale, where it releases as you exhale.

Your breathing pattern may vary at different points of the day. It may also change according to your mood, previous activity and current thoughts. Many factors contribute to what you find as you simply relax and observe.

Feel the interior spaces as your breath enters your head and begins its interior journey down through your trachea into your lungs. Notice where you feel the natural motions of your breathing. Does it feel labored or effortless? Do you notice one target area receiving the breath more than some other regions? Can you distinguish a temperature difference between the inhalation and the exhalation as it moves through your nostrils?

Let your awareness now focus on your abdominal region and allow a gentle expansion there as you inhale. Now, let the area contract and sink inward as you exhale. If this is different from your normal breath, place your hands on your lower abdomen and gently compress your abdominal muscles as you exhale. This breath awareness is for the purpose of concentrating your attention and toning your abdominal muscles. While the effort is mild, over time it will definitely tone your abdominals with its wave-like motions.

When you sustain this directing of the breath while lying down, it naturally stimulates a relaxation reflex. In reaction to this normal parasympathetic reflex, your respiratory rate will diminish, your heart rate will lower and elevated blood pressure will begin to normalize. This comes about through a neurological sensor called the baroreceptor located on the wall of the descending aorta. This reflex is activated when pressure is applied to the middle abdomen during exhalation. The pressure change is sensed by the baroreceptor, which, in turn, signals the hypothalamus in the mid-brain. The hypothalamus is responsible for regulating heart rate and blood pressure. The tension of the arterial wall tells the system that less pressure is needed in the system, which causes the blood pressure and heart rate to be lowered. Once you can create these abdominal waves at will, you will find this to be an effective method to relax, regardless of what activity you may be engaged in.

To begin the process of breath awareness, observe the nature of your breathing pattern while visualizing your respiratory system.

Inhale: Your diaphragm goes down as air rushes into your lungs. The action of the diaphragm widens your rib cage and also pushes your abdominal contents downward and forward.

Exhale: Your diaphragm returns to its original position, and air is expelled from your lungs. Your abdomen draws in and up when you breathe out.

It is important to note that, for about half the population, this is not a normal event. The other half of the world breathes in reverse of this description. That is, they swell the belly during exhalation and expand the chest during inhalation. The belly contracts during inhalation and the chest relaxes during exhalation. This reverse breathing is due to the exaggerated use of the chest, neck and shoulders. Accompanying this respiratory pattern are often chronic tension in the neck and shoulders and irregular biological rhythms—menstrual flow, constipation, frequent or evening urination, insomnia, elevated blood pressure and even tachycardia (irregular heart rhythms).

It has been my consistent experience that when people regain this natural pattern, some of the most obvious symptoms of stress in their lives begin to fade away. So simple, yet so complex. This is the biological reflex of the life-force coming into and from the human body. To make this shift requires some patience and perseverance that is well worth the benefits you will experience.

Not convinced? Next time you are stressed out, check out your breathing and see how it is moving. I guarantee that the wave pattern is not present if you feel tense. Change your breath and allow any other change to follow from that. In summary, the natural breathing pattern in yoga practice is wave-like, moving through the nostrils as follows:

To breathe in: expand your chest first and then let your breath descend like a wave to your lower abdomen.

To breathe out: allow your abdomen to go in, pulling in and up on your musculature, then let the wave return upward.

## How Breathing Affects Posture

The way breathing affects posture and the way posture affects breathing is complementary. The importance of these issues has long been recognized in yoga, but most commentaries are vague and imprecise. Here, I am aiming for simplicity: photographic records of exhalations and inhalations and superimpositions of computer-generated tracings of inhalations (since these are always larger) on the exhalations. The single most important key to understanding all such effects is the operation of the respiratory diaphragm, and to introduce the subject, we'll explore 2 exercises that will help you become aware of its anatomy and understand 2 of its main roles in movement, other than respiration itself.

### A variation of the Cobra Pose

Lie face down on the floor and interlock your arms behind your back, grasping your forearms or elbows. Or you can simply place your hands in the standard cobra position alongside the chest. Strongly tighten all the muscles from the hips to the toes, and use the neck and deep back muscles to lift the head, neck and chest as high as possible. You are not making any particular use of the diaphragm to come into this position. Now, inhale and exhale deeply through the nose. Notice that each inhalation raises the upper part of the body higher and that each exhalation lowers it. Because you are keeping the back muscles engaged continuously during both inhalation and exhalation, the lifting and lowering action is due entirely to the muscles of respiration. In this variation of the Cobra Pose, we hold the hips, thighs and pelvis firmly, which stabilizes the lower back and the spinal attachment of the crus of the diaphragm. Inhalation creates tension at all three of the diaphragm's attachments: one on the vertebral column, one on the base of the rib cage and the third on the central tendon. But because the hip and thigh muscles have been tightened, the spinal attachment is stabilized, except a slight lifting effect that is translated to the hips. What happens in the torso illustrates clearly how respiratory movements influence posture: with the abdomen pressed against the floor, the contents of the abdominal cavity cannot easily descend, and this restricts the downward movement of the central tendon, which now acts as a link between the 2 muscular portions of the diaphragm. With the crural attachments stabilized, the only insertion that can be mobilized without difficulty is the one at the base of the rib cage. This attachment therefore expands the chest from its base, draws air into the lungs, and lifts the upper body. If you are breathing smoothly and deeply you will feel a gentle, rhythmic rocking movement as the head, neck, and chest rise and fall with each inhalation and exhalation. This is a perfect illustration of thoraco-diaphragmatic breathing. In this exercise, the action of the diaphragm during inhalation reinforces the activity of the deep back and neck muscles and thus deepens the backward bend. During exhalation, the muscle fibers of the diaphragm lengthen eccentrically as they resist gravity. When they finally relax at the end of exhalation, the backward bend in the spine is maintained only by the deep muscles of the back and neck. This is an excellent exercise for strengthening the diaphragm, because after you have lifted to your maximum with the deep back muscles, you are using the diaphragm, aided by the external intercostal muscles acting as synergists, to raise the upper half of the body even higher—and this is a substantial mass to be lifted by a single sheet of muscle acting as prime mover. Furthermore, if you keep trying as hard as possible to inhale deeply without closing the glottis, you will be creating the most extreme possible isometric exercise for this muscle and its synergists, the external intercostals.

## The Diaphragmatic Rear Lift

Next, try a posture that we can aptly call the diaphragmatic rear lift. Again, lie face down, placing your chin against the floor, with the arms along the sides of the body and the palms next to the chest. Keeping the chest pressed firmly against the floor, relax all the muscles from the waist down, including the hips. Take 10–15 nasal breaths at a rate of about one breath per second. With the thighs and hips relaxed, and with the base of the rib cage fixed against the floor, the action of the diaphragm during inhalation can be translated to only one site: the spinal attachment of the crus. And because the deep back muscles are relaxed, each inhalation lifts the lower back and hips, and each exhalation allows them to fall toward the floor. Make sure you produce the movement entirely with the diaphragm, not by bumping your hips up and down with the gluteal (hip) and back muscles. Because the inhalations increase the lumbar curvature, this exercise will not be comfortable for anyone with lower back pain.

If the gluteal region and lower extremities remain completely relaxed, the crural attachments of the diaphragm then lift the hips during inhalation and lower them back down during exhalation.

You can feel the diaphragmatic rear lift most easily if you breathe rapidly; the quick inhalations whip the hips up and away from the floor and the sudden exhalations drop them. But if you breathe slowly and smoothly, you will notice that each inhalation gradually increases the pull and tension on the hips and lower back, even though it does not create much movement, and that each exhalation gradually eases the tension. When you are breathing slowly enough, you can also feel the muscle fibers of the diaphragm shorten concentrically during inhalation and lengthen eccentrically during exhalation as they control the gravity induced lowering of the hips toward the floor.

The origins and insertions of the diaphragm are reversed in the diaphragmatic rear lift in comparison with the cobra variation, and this creates repercussions throughout the whole body. In the cobra variation, we fix the hips and thighs, allowing the costal attachment of the diaphragm to lift the rib cage and with it, the entire upper half of the body. In the diaphragmatic rear lift we do just the opposite: we fix the rib cage, relax the hips and thighs, and allow the crural insertion of the diaphragm to lift the lumbar spine and hips.

These 2 postures also show us how important it is that the diaphragm is indented so deeply by the vertebral column that it almost encircles the spine. This enables it to act both from above and behind to accentuate the lumbar arch during inhalation, lifting the upper half of the body in the cobra variation, and lifting the sacrum and hips in the diaphragmatic rear lift.

## *Anatomy of Natural Respiration*

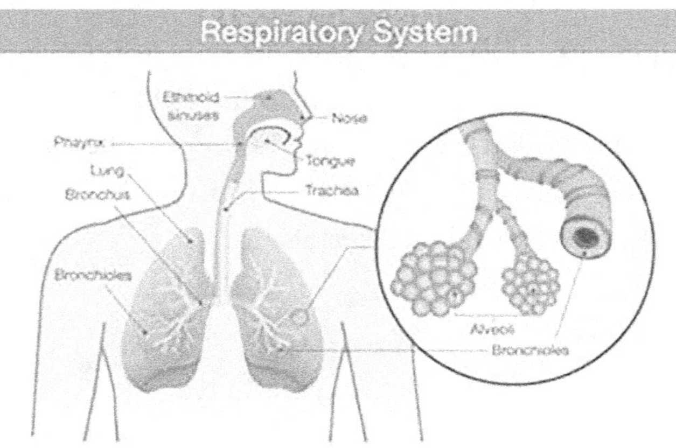


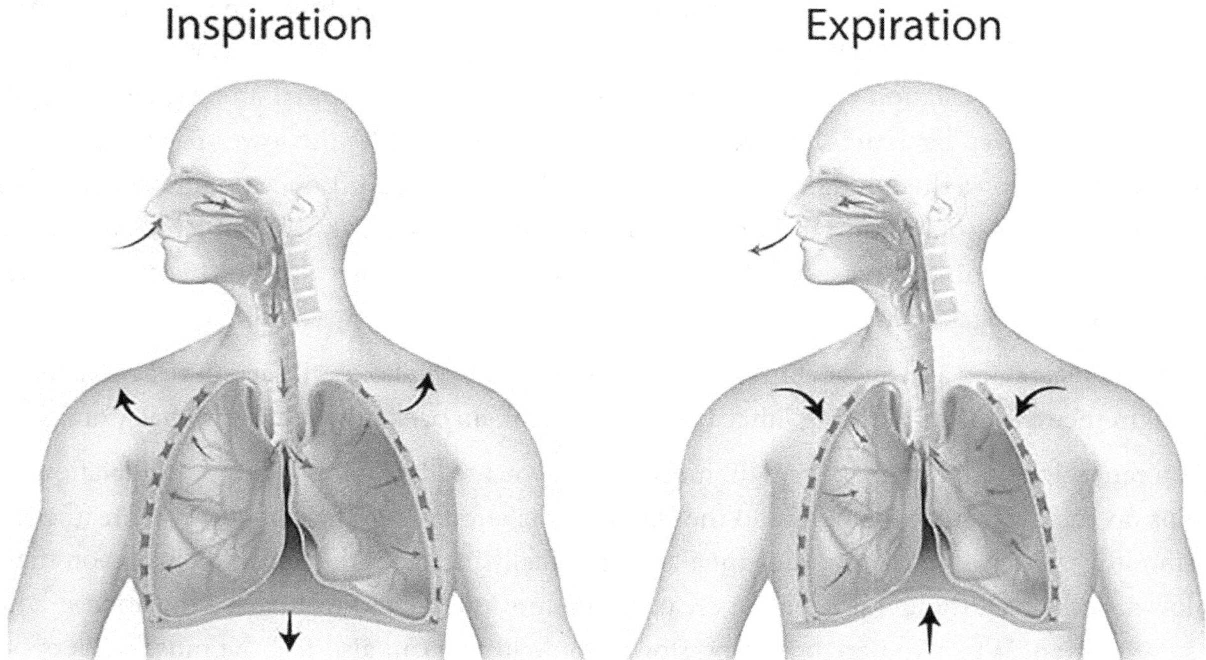


As you inhale, the large muscle of the diaphragm moves down, flattening out as it goes, causing the lower ribs to expand and the abdominal organs to move down and forward. Natural inhalation acts as a massage to the upper abdominal organs—liver, stomach, large intestine and pancreas. A full normal inhalation will massage even the mid-abdominal organs—the ascending and descending large intestine and the centrally located small intestines. The abdominal muscles must relax for this to occur. Thus, there is a slight swelling of the belly from top to bottom, giving the appearance of a wave-like motion.

During normal exhalation, the diaphragm is moved up and the lungs are collapsed. With yoga training, the contractions will be felt like a reverse wave from the bottom of the abdomen toward the chest. This action is made possible by toning the centrally located rectus abdominis muscle. It is assisted in breathing by the tone of the lateral abdominals, the abdominus oblique internus and externus and the abdominus lateralis. During full expiration, the diaphragm relaxes back to a dome shape, mildly compressing the lungs and heart, while narrowing the rib cage. The rib movements are caused by 2 sets of muscles between the ribs: the internal and external inter-costal. These muscles depress and narrow the rib cage during exhalation, while in inhalation they reverse the process to expand the rib cage's diameter, thereby increasing the internal cavity space to allow the lungs to open.

During normal breath training, these sets of muscles—the diaphragm, rectus abdominis and the 2 sets of inter-costal—are strengthened and trained to move more air in and out. This increases the quantity of circulating air within the body (called the tidal volume—500ml) and diminishes the number of breaths per minute (normal rate of respiration in adults is 12–20 breaths per minute). It requires both practice and heightened awareness to train your respiratory motions. With persistence, the breath can stimulate circulation to the kidneys, spleen and the adrenal glands located in the middle back. A good way to begin is to rest in a prone position—like the Crocodile (Makarasana) or the Fetal Pose—and direct the breath to your lower back. In both these positions, the lower back is mildly stretched during inhalation. By deepening your breath to your back, the diaphragm is encouraged to extend downward, which, in turn, can facilitate the opening of the lower lobes of the lung.

## The Nostrils and Wind Pipe

Most yoga breathing exercises (pranayama) are done by drawing air in through the nostrils. The nostrils are lined with mucous membranes that serve to moisten the air and filter out any heavy particles that get trapped and may be toxic to the internal organs. The nostrils are also lined with small hair follicles that act to change the direction of the airflow and heighten its speed. As the breath passes the nose, it enters a series of pathways called the superior, middle and inferior meatus and the superior, middle and inferior concha. These structures act like turbines to increase the speed and direct the flow of the breath toward the deeper lobes of the lungs. They also permit warming of the air immediately before entering the pharynx en route to the trachea. In contrast, with mouth breathing, the mucous membranes in the throat dry out, increasing the risk of irritation and infection. Notice the difference in yourself between mouth and nostril breathing.

Which one can you sustain?

Which one feels most natural?

Breathing through the nose also stimulates the olfactory nerves, heightening sensations of aroma. Our sense of smell is connected to the earth element, according to Ayurveda. This element creates our sense of groundedness, a connection with gravity and the Earth.

## The Lungs

The anatomy of the lungs is fascinating. They are pear shaped, with small upper lobes capable of containing only about ½ cup of air each. The lower lungs can contain about 1¼ quarts of air. The upper lobes extend above the collarbones and can be palpated by applying pressure at the sides of the neck, where the neck joins the clavicles. The lower lungs are wider than the upper lungs when viewed from the front, and they fill the entire width of the middle rib cage. The bottoms of the lungs are concave, conforming to the shape of the diaphragm's dome.

## The Diaphragm and Intercostals

The major muscle of respiration is the diaphragm. This large flat muscle is shaped somewhat like a full parachute or a dome. It fills the entire inner circumference below the lungs and heart, attaching to the rib cage and lumbar spine. It serves to divide the vital organs resting above it, from the digestive organs that reside below it. The diaphragm's motion is similar to that of a piston, just as the lungs are similar to a combustion chamber. When the diaphragm contracts, it moves downward, pulling air inward with the inhaling motion. Its contraction transforms its shape from a lofty dome to something rather like a Frisbee saucer that has widened in its downward motion. During normal breathing, the motion is rather shallow. Hence, air does not enter the lungs' larger lower regions. With a full inhalation, air reaches into the lower lungs, where there is more space to receive the full capacity of respiration. The blood supply to the lower lobes is gravity dependent, so when we are upright there is far more blood available for oxygen exchange in the lower parts of the lungs. It is for this reason that diaphragmatic breathing, which draws air into those lower regions, is such an essential component of optimal exercise breathing.

In the yoga breathing practices, the diaphragm is contracted and lowered on the inhale, with the abdominal muscles controlled, so that the breath is drawn in slowly and consciously. "The combined action of the diaphragm and the abdominal muscles pulls up the lower part of the spinal column… This pulling up of the vertebral column as a whole, gives exercise to the sympathetic and the roots of the spinal nerves." During exhalation, the diaphragm relaxes upward, which allows for the release of carbon dioxide and other metabolic waste gases. At this time, the diaphragm relaxes back to its dome shape, mildly compressing the lungs and heart while narrowing the rib cage. The rib motions are caused by 2 sets of muscles located between the ribs, the internal and external intercostal. These muscles open and elevate the ribs to expand the circumference and increase the internal cavity for the lungs during inhalation. The muscles contract in reverse during the exhale.

With yoga breathing, these three sets of muscles, the diaphragm and the intercostals, are strengthened to such an extent that more air is moved in and out during a normal respiratory cycle. Thus, the effects of pranayama training last throughout the day. This increases the quantity of circulating air (called the tidal volume) and diminishes the number of breaths per minute. The net effect is a more efficient respiratory apparatus.

The piston engine of an automobile is similar in design to the respiratory system. When the piston goes down, it pulls air into the chamber above it. This action intensifies the pressure in the combustion chamber, located above the piston. When the piston rises, it forces air out, creating a strong burst of energy to be released to your car's drivetrain. The major difference in this analogy is that, unlike a car's cylinder, your rib cage has the capacity to expand with the downward piston-like motion of the diaphragm. This additional dimension of motion allows for the possibility of tremendously increased power and vitality.

## Diaphragmatic and Abdominal Breathing

Begin breath training by watching the breath as you inhale and exaggerating the expansion caused by the downward motion of your diaphragm. Place your hands on your abdomen at or below your navel. You will notice the lower abdomen gently swell during inhalation. A common misconception is that diaphragmatic breathing differs from abdominal. In yoga training, they flow one into the other. By emphasizing one, different benefits arise. Some people are under the mistaken impression that this breathing motion will decrease abdominal muscle tone. Nothing could be farther from the truth. In yoga breath training, we emphasize relaxation during inhalation and controlled toning of the abdominals during exhalation. The control comes primarily from toning the large vertical central muscle, the rectus abdominis.

Breathing focused on just this region has a sedative effect if done for a 2 to 10 minute cycle. It helps you relax as it reduces blood pressure and respiratory rate. If done regularly, it can be developed into a tool to help you fall asleep more rapidly. It is a really important breathing pattern to master as it is a tool you will need for stressful periods of life. When you can accomplish it in an active standing position, you will be able to apply it during a stressful conversation to help relieve the physical tension accompanying your impatience or anxiety.

A variation is to breathe through your mouth with a sighing sound. By allowing an audible sound to escape, you can deepen the discharge of stress. You will probably note that you have done this in the past. Indeed, sighing is natural, as you release a stressful event. By training the sigh to become prolonged and audible, you can make yourself more effective at putting the event into a discriminating perspective. This breathing is not recommended except for short periods of time. Do not continue it more than five minutes unless you are ready to sleep.

## The Wave Pattern

Breathing exercises are in wave motion. This is a continuation of the diaphragmatic and abdominal breath in which a greater amount of air can be taken in when respiratory motions extend among three regions—the lower abdomen, solar plexus and the chest.

During inhalation, your chest expands naturally first, then the expansion progresses to the lower ribs and lastly into the abdomen. The inhalation is essentially a descending vertical motion. With this descent, the lower rib cage widens and the upper abdominal organs are displaced downward and forward. As in the abdominal breath, there is a mild expansion of the abdomen at the end of the inhalation.

The exhalation is the reverse of the inhalation. Its motion is an ascending vertical flow of breath. It begins with a mild contraction in the lower abdominal muscles to propel the exhaled air from the bottom of the lungs. During the mid-range of exhalation, the lower rib cage narrows to promote the ascent of the diaphragm. This is the natural manner of breathing that coordinates the functioning of all the respiratory structures and musculature.

The desired effect is an evenness of motion in all four portions of the body—chest, rib cage, diaphragm and abdomen. This exercise requires you to be motionless in order to feel the effect. Thus, it is best learned in a seated or supine position. The complete exercise moves all the respiratory muscles to full capacity in a passive manner, preventing stress to the heart and autonomic nervous system. If your breath expansion is too great in the upper region, this causes the clavicle bone to rise and stimulate your heart rate and blood pressure. This is the breath pattern predominant in people who have heart conditions or asthma. Changing their breathing pattern may lessen the underlying physical and emotional tensions.

Next, turn your attention inward and notice the quality of your breath. Allow your breath to become a natural wave that moves up and down your interior body. Ideally, it will become smooth and constant with no pause, an inhalation and exhalation of equal length. Maintain a consistent rhythm, full and deep, feeling more internal than external motion. The breathing cycle should be slowed to 8 to 10 breaths per minute, rather than the average 12 to 15 per minute. Breathing should be silent to others, making a nasal sound audible only to the practitioner. Your nostrils should not flare during the cycle. Your lower jaw should be relaxed, with your teeth slightly separated. In general, allow your face to be relaxed with a serene expression.

Once you understand—and feel—the anatomy of breathing, you will be able to move on to the subtler components of the breath. Unlike the abdominal breath, the complete wave breath is not sedative. Rather, it is an invigorating breath that brings your body to rest, while simultaneously promoting mental clarity.

## Ujjayi Breathing

Your next breathing tool is Ujjayi Breathing. Ujjayi comes from 2 root words, uj, meaning "upward," and jayi, meaning "victorious." It is a breathing technique that helps the mind rise victoriously above its usually restless nature to experience the Self. The mind then becomes calm, and the stillness that is always there beneath your thoughts shines clear, giving an experience of your inner Self. An important technique for Hatha Yoga, ujjayi is a glottal breath in which the glottis at the back of the throat is partially closed to narrow the passage of air entering from the sinus cavities and nostrils to the trachea (wind pipe).

Ujjayi is the basic pranayama technique from which most others derive. It is best done seated in a chair or in a meditation pose, with your back erect and your head slightly down, as in bowing toward your heart. The chest/heart is raised to allow the lungs freedom to expand easily. Place your hands, palm up, on your knees with the tips of your forefinger and thumbs joined in Jnana Mudra (Wisdom's Seal) and your arms straight. Place your attention on the breath sound. Maintain inhalation and exhalation at an even, steady pace. Create a constriction in the base of your throat that makes the sound more audible. Begin by taking a deep breath and feel the soft juncture above and between your collarbones (clavicles) where the breast bone (sternum) sinks in. It is this contraction that creates the breath sound. The sound should be evenly made from the beginning to the end of each inhalation and each exhalation. Don't pause while breathing, but maintain a smooth, steady in-out flowing cycle. When this has been stable for 5 minutes, you may begin the second phase of practice, extending the natural length of each breath. This follows with the second definition of pranayama. Drawing out the breath deepens your ability to concentrate and maintain a still posture. Your breath becomes subtler, the prana energy in the breath more apparent. The influence of the mind becomes more obvious.

The breath is said to create the natural mantra sound of hamsa. Ham is the sound of the inhalation, sa the sound of exhalation. The mantra means, "I am that." The "that" refers to pure awareness. In this way, breath can be used as a meditation device to attract your mind. You may become aware of "ham" on inhale and "sa" on exhale. By gently keeping your mind on this awareness, the process of meditation spontaneously arises from within. Deepen this process by practicing regularly.

## Variations

There are numerous variations of this practice that alter the ratio of inhalation to exhalation, add breath pauses (Kumbhaka) or alternate the nostril through which you breathe. These practices are best learned directly from a teacher and hence will not be covered here.

## Benefit

Ujjayi is excellent for respiratory patients, especially asthmatics. When regularly practiced, it is an excellent doorway into natural meditation.

## Using Breath in Asana Practice

One of the hallmarks of Classical Yoga is the consistent use of ujjayi pranayama (in the wave motion) in asana practice. This feature and the development of breathing exercises into pranayama, which enlivens the life-force, make Classical Yoga unique as a personal discipline.

In asana practice, there are three general rules for the use of breath patterns.

1.  Inhalation occurs as you extend the spine, exhalation when you release tension and relax.

    Rhythmic breath is harmonized to be at the pace of body motions. For example, if I am in an erect standing position (Tadasana) and I lift my arms up, I inhale during this motion. With practice, I can learn to pace the tempo of my arms' motions with the time required to fill my lungs. In this manner, the inhalation will be complete when the arms reach full shoulder flexion, fingertips aimed at the ceiling. Similarly, I can exhale to lower my arms to my sides and I run out of breath when my arms touch my sides.

2.  Inhale when you move to center or become erect and exhale when moving away from the centered position. Bending forward is to be accompanied by an exhalation. Sitting up can accompany an inhalation. Twisting or side bending can be done with an exhalation, while returning to centered erect posture can occur on an inhalation. If I move slowly into a forwarding position, I extend myself, lengthening my spine with each inhalation, and moving forward with each exhalation.

3.  Breath awareness is constant, even when your body is stationary. When I hold an asana, my attention remains on the internal wavelike flow of ujjayi. If my intention is to deepen the physical pose by continually going into a wider range of motion, my breath can be used to release specific tension areas that restrict my breath or body sensations, wherever they may be. In this procedure, revert to the first rule and notice that your body continues to lengthen itself during inhalation. A keen concentration will uncover where the opening is taking place. On the next inhalation, gently move yourself in the pattern revealed by the openness of your breath. On the next exhalation, release the tension, observing carefully where and in what direction the release takes place. This will guide you to move on the next inhalation. Once you have reached the boundary of this openness, you can choose between staying at the new edge of your pose or inhaling on your way back to a centered position. The qualities of the breath are intriguing to examine. Classical Yoga regulates all 4 pans of the breath—the 2 motions (inhalation and exhalation) and the 2 pauses that naturally follow the motions. The pauses are natural, provided

there is no stress or fixed attention. During either of these events, the natural rhythm is altered and the breath will be shallower and the pauses longer. A major difference between stress and concentration is that the pause during stress is accompanied by effort and tension, and it increases internal pressure. With concentration, the pause is a natural and effortless event. Upon closer examination, the breath is not held nor does it stop. Rather it persists with subtle, nearly imperceptible, waves. Provided your concentration is genuine, do not encourage yourself to breathe deeply during yoga asana practice. Only if you are exhibiting holding your breath should you be encouraged to breathe fully. Watching carefully for this distinction can permit you to move into a deeper connection with the process of Classical Yoga. It is often a missing link, a hidden secret, that practitioners disregard in learning how to transition from physical Hatha Yoga to mindful Raja Yoga practice.

## How Long to Hold a Pose

Based upon the breath patterns, there are different benefits for holding poses at varying lengths.

1. Inhale into the pose, exhale to release the pose.

   This pattern is useful for becoming familiar with the movement and how your body reacts. By repeated practice in this manner, sensitivity is heightened and your body will uncover its own homeostasis. When this method is repeated for up to 6 times, it is optimal for slowing down your mind, deepening your breath and developing pranic energy. It is a form of pranayama that regulates the flow of prana into the areas of the body affected by the asana.

2. Staying in the pose for 2 to 3 breaths.

   This pattern is useful for training concentration (dhyana) and integrating pranayama ratios into asana. It is particularly beneficial for improving memory, gently strengthening the lungs and for students with scoliosis. At this level of concentration, 2 points of anatomical alignment may be maintained, but the practice is not for developing detailed body posturing. When this method is repeated, it heightens the body's ability to adapt, thus improving efficiency in eliminating stress and hypertension.

3. Staying in the posture for 12 breaths.

   This is the level I recommend for optimizing the effects of muscular strength or flexibility for those students who are focusing on eliminating specific muscular and postural imbalances. This develops optimal stamina in the shortest possible period. To proceed, begin by holding the pose with good alignment and steadiness at a lesser number of breaths, then increase the holding time by 2 to 3 breaths per week. When the posture can be held comfortably and steadily for 12 breaths for 2 weeks consistently, you can move on to the next level of challenge.

## The Dangers of Holding Your Breath

"It is dangerous to hold your breath during any form of exercise," writes Michael O'Shea.

"As you inhale and exhale, the pressure in your chest cavity increases and decreases. When you exercise and are breathing heavier, these pressure changes are even greater. When you hold your breath, you do not allow for the natural release of this pressure, and the stress on your heart and circulatory system can elevate blood pressure two to three times above normal. This can result in ruptured blood vessels, stroke or heart attack." In yoga practice, as in any unfamiliar activity, it is common to hold your breath due to the concentration involved. This should not be encouraged. For beginners, one major value of a teacher is to encourage full conscious respiration during all yoga activities. Once the student has spent about a year with the practice, there are exercises that can be given to allow for the natural pause between respiratory motions to be gently increased. This practice should be supervised and, in general, done only with the coordination of muscular locks to regulate blood pressure and heart rate. The side effects cited above can be alleviated with proper supervision. In general, however, it is advisable not to hold your breath during yoga practices of asana or pranayama. The muscular locks (bandhas) may appear easy to learn, but their proper development requires physical supervision by a teacher trained in their physical and energetic benefits.

## Bandha

We will now try to understand in detail the second aspect of the basic fundamentals of asana practice, that is, Bandha.

Bandhas are "locks" occurring throughout the body. A combination of opposing muscles forms these locks, stimulating nerve conduction and illuminating the chakras.

All the three diaphragms (pelvic, respiratory and vocal) plus ujjayi come together in yoga movements that are coordinated with inhalation and exhalation. In addition to giving more length and texture to the breath, the "valve" of ujjayi creates a kind of back pressure throughout the abdominal and thoracic cavities that can increase the flexibility of the spine during the long, slow flexion and extension movements that occur in vinyasas such as the sun salutations.

In yogic terms, these actions of the diaphragms (bandhas) create more sthira (stability) in the body, protecting it from injury by redistributing mechanical stress. An additional effect of moving the body through this resistance is the creation of heat in the system, which can be used in many beneficial ways. These practices are referred to as brahmana, which implies heat, expansion and the development of power and strength as well as the ability to withstand stress. Brahmana is also associated with inhaling, nourishment, prana and the chest region. When relaxing the body in the more supported, horizontal, restorative practices, remember to release the bandhas and glottal constrictions that are associated with vertical postural support. This relaxing side of yoga embodies the qualities of langhana, which is associated with coolness, condensation, relaxation and release as well as the development of sensitivity and inward focus. Langhana is also associated with exhaling, elimination of apana (one among five types of vatha or intestinal gas) and the abdominal region. Because the ultimate goal of yoga breath training is to free up the system from habitual, dysfunctional restrictions, the first thing you need to do is free yourself from the idea that there's a single right way to breathe. As useful as the bandhas are when supporting your center of gravity and moving the spine through space, you need to release the forces of sthira in the system when pursuing the relaxation and release of sukha. If yoga practice leads you to more integrated, balanced breathing, it's because it trains your body to freely respond to the demands that you place on it in the various positions and activities that make up your daily life.

In hatha yoga, the pelvic diaphragm is activated consciously by 2 practices: Ashwini Mudra and Mula Bandha. The 2 have subtle and not-so-subtle differences. We'll begin with Ashwini Mudra.

**Ashwini Mudra:** Ashwini is the Sanskrit word for "mare" and Ashwini Mudra in hatha yoga is named for the movement of the pelvic diaphragm in a horse after it has expelled the contents of its bowel.

During the expulsion phase, the cone-shaped pelvic diaphragm moves to the rear, and after the contents of the bowel are dropped, the muscles of the pelvic diaphragm pull strongly inward. In so doing they cleanse the anal canal. In human beings, the same thing happens—you first bear down, opening the anus and expelling the contents of the bowel, and then the pelvic diaphragm pulls inward and upward while contracting the anal sphincter. The pulling inward motion, which we also do reflexively from moment to moment during the day, is Ashwini Mudra. This is not as obvious as it is in a horse, because in humans the whole region is enveloped in loose connective tissue and covered with the superficial structures of the perineum, but it is the same gesture.

As a natural movement, Ashwini Mudra is often forceful, especially when it is associated with keeping the base of the abdominopelvic cavity sealed during sharp or extreme increases in intra-abdominal pressure or when it is used as a last-ditch means for retention (think of restraining diarrhea).

As a yoga practice, Ashwini Mudra is not so intense, but it still acts as a perianal seal, fortified in this case by tightening the gluteal muscles along with the pelvic diaphragm and anal sphincter. The mudra is applied for a few seconds, released and repeated. Ideally, only the gluteals, the pelvic diaphragm and the anal sphincter are activated, but the proximity of muscles overlying the genitals anteriorly sometimes makes this difficult, and you will often feel them tighten along with the rest when you try to create the gesture.

Some postures make a pure Ashwini Mudra easy, and others make it difficult. If you stand with the feet well apart and bend forward 20–30°, you will find it awkward to contract the anus and pelvic diaphragm and almost impossible to contract them without activating the muscles around the genitals as well.

Now stand upright with the heels and toes together and try it again. This is easier. If you don't tighten too vigorously you may be able to isolate the pelvic diaphragm and the gluteals from the muscles of the genitals. Next, bend backward gently, keeping the heels together and the thighs rotated out so the feet are pointed 90° away from one another. Keep the knees extended. Then, gently tighten behind and try to release in front. This is one of the easiest upright postures in which to accomplish a pure Ashwini Mudra. Last, bring the toes together and rotate the heels out. This again makes it difficult. These simple experiments illustrate the general rule: any posture that pulls the hips together will make Ashwini Mudra easier, and any posture that pulls the hips apart will make it more difficult. That, as it happens, is one problem with all cross-legged sitting postures. Try it. When the thighs are flexed with respect to the spine and abducted out to the sides, it is almost impossible to contract the gluteal and only a little less difficult to isolate the anus and pelvic diaphragm from the genitals. But if you try the mudra in the shoulder stand or headstand with the heels together and the toes out, you will find that it is easy because gravity is already pulling the pelvic diaphragm toward the floor. Little or no effort is needed to achieve a fully pulled-in feeling, and that effort need not involve the genitals. Now lie supine on the floor and notice that you can easily tighten up in the rear without recruiting muscles around the genitals. Prone, it is more difficult, at least in men, in whom the muscles associated with the genitals are stimulated by contact with the floor. One of the best postures for Ashwini Mudra is the Upward-Facing Dog. As long as the pelvis is lifted slightly off the floor, it is impossible to do this pose without activating the pelvic diaphragm, yet it does not stimulate the muscles in the urogenital triangle in the least. The Downward-Facing Dog, not surprisingly, creates the opposite effect: this posture is one of the easiest poses for recruiting the muscles of the urogenital region in isolation, but a pose in which it is almost impossible to isolate the muscles associated with Ashwini Mudra.

## Mula Bandha, the Root Lock

Unlike Ashwini Mudra, which is often a response to sharp and sudden increases in abdominopelvic pressure, Mula Bandha (the root lock) is a gentle contraction of the pelvic diaphragm and the muscles of the urogenital triangle. It does not counter intra-abdominal pressure so much as it seals urogenital energy within the body, controlling and restraining it during breathing exercises and meditation (again, this is a literary rather than a scientific use of the term "energy"). What actually happens is more easily sensed than described, so we'll begin with a series of exercises.

First try sitting in a hard chair covered with a thin cushion. In a neutral position, neither perfectly upright or slumped, try to blow out but without letting any air escape. Try hard. Notice that the pelvic region contracts and lifts up involuntarily enough to counter the downward push from the chest and abdominal wall. Now try the mock blowing maneuver again, but this time keep the pelvic region relaxed, and notice that it feels like straining for a bowel movement. Try it one last time, but this time lift the entire anatomical perineum consciously, and you will quickly sense that these efforts bring both the pelvic diaphragm and the muscles of the urogenital region into play.

Next sit really straight, arching the lower back forward. Exhale, pressing in with the abdominal muscles, and notice that it is natural to find a focus for your attention at a point between the anus and genitals. You may sense a slight tension in the muscles of the genitals, but little or none in the anus, and certainly none in the gluteal muscles. This describes the root lock. You don't have to make extreme efforts. The cushion on which you are sitting places enough pressure on the muscles of the urogenital triangle to focus your awareness on the lock.

Now try the same exercise in a slumped posture with the back rounded to the rear. This changes everything. It shifts your attention from the front of the anatomical perineum to the rear, and it elicits a mild Ashwini Mudra instead of Mula Bandha because you are tipping backward toward the plane of the anal triangle and away from the plane of the urogenital triangle. Sitting straight rocks you up and forward so that contact with the cushion favors the root lock. The lesson: sit straight if you wish to apply Mula Bandha.

If this is still confusing, it will be helpful to first experience a gross version of the root lock. The best concentration exercise for this is to sit upright and try breathing in concert with slowly increasing and decreasing tension in the perineum. With the beginning of exhalation gradually tighten the muscles of the pelvic diaphragm and genitals, aiming for maximum contraction at the end of exhalation.

As inhalation begins, slowly relax. Repeat the cycle for 10 breaths several times a day. At first, it may be difficult to tighten the muscles without also tightening the gluteal muscles, but if you are careful to sit straight it will become easy.

With practice, you will be able to sense the contraction of successive layers of muscles from the outside in. Starting superficially and with minimal effort, you can feel activity in the ischiocavernosus, bulbospongiosus and superficial transverse perineal muscles. With a little more attention, you can activate the deep transverse perineal muscles and the urethral sphincter. With yet more effort, you can activate the pelvic diaphragm. The central tendon of the perineum, which, as discussed previously, is located at the dividing line between the anal and urogenital triangles, appears to be the key structure around which the more delicate versions of Mula Bandha are organized. This is an extremely tough fascial region into which the superficial and deep transverse perineal muscles insert. If you can learn to focus your attention on this tiny region while creating minimal physical contraction of the nearby muscles, you will be feeling the root lock. (Yoga teachers who speak of placing awareness on the perineum are referring to this region.) Concentrate on the sensation, and in time, Mula Bandha will feel natural and comfortable. With experience, you can hold the lock constantly, which is what yogis recommend for meditation.

In Ashwini Mudra, we strongly activate the pelvic diaphragm, the anus and the gluteals. Mula Bandha is more delicate. Here, we mildly activate the pelvic diaphragm plus—more strongly—the overlying muscles of the urogenital triangle, which includes the muscles associated with the genitals and the urethra. Therefore, to understand Mula Bandha, we must examine the anatomical disposition of these muscles.

## *The Muscles of the Urogenital Triangle (Perineal Muscles)*

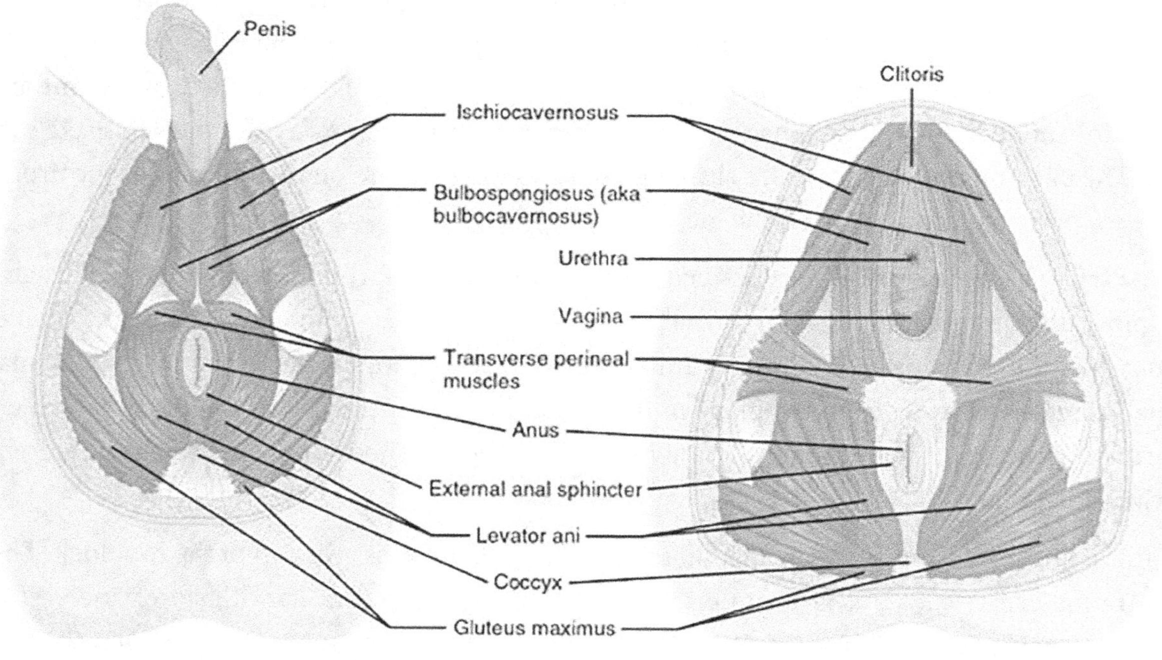


Male perineal muscles: inferior view

Female perineal muscles: inferior view

Looking at a superficial dissection, we see that three pairs of muscles overlie the genitals. In both male and female, the superficial transverse perineal muscles course laterally in the shared border of the urogenital and anal triangles, extending laterally from a heavy band of centrally located connective tissue—the central tendon of the perineum—to the ischial tuberosities. The bulbospongiosus muscles in the male encircle the base of the penis; in the female, those same muscles encircle the vagina and urethra. The ischiocavernosus muscles in both the male and female lie superficial to the erectile tissues of the corpora cavernosa, which course from the inferior pubic rami to the body of the penis in the male and to the clitoris in the female. In a slightly deeper plane of the urogenital diaphragm (in both male and female), the deep transverse perineal muscles spread out laterally in sheets that attach to the inferior pubic rami, and the urethral sphincters encircle the urethrae.

## A modified Cat Stretch

In addition to the Downward-Facing Dog, which was mentioned in the section on Ashwini Mudra, one of the best yoga postures for helping you come in contact with the delicacy and precision of the root lock is a modified Cat Pose. From a kneeling position, bring your chin to the floor, swing your elbows out and bring the upper part of the chest as low as possible, arching your back deeply and mimicking a cat peering under a couch. Then tighten the perianal region generally. You will immediately notice that the exposed anus in this position brings the sensations toward the front of the diamond-shaped perineum rather than behind, and that even if you squeeze vigorously the gluteal muscles remain relaxed. After you have practiced this pose several times and got accustomed to its associated sensations, you can try to find the same feelings when you apply the root lock in sitting postures.

## Agni Sara

Agni Sara, or "fanning the fire," is a breathing exercise, an abdominal exercise and a powerful stimulus to abdomino-pelvic health. When it is done with full attention and for an adequate span of daily practice, it stokes the fire of the body like no other exercise. But before trying it, we'll first do a training exercise for active exhalations and then work with a moderate practice—A and P breathing—that is accessible to everyone.

## Active Exhalation

During relaxed, casual breathing, you make moderate efforts to inhale and you usually relax to exhale, but all the exercises that follow make use of active exhalations, in some cases breathing out all the way down to your residual volume.

To get an idea of what is involved, try the following exercise: Inhale moderately through the nose, purse the lips and exhale as if you were trying to blow up a balloon in one breath. Try this several times. If you slowly breathe out as much air as possible through the resistance of the pursed lips, you'll notice that exhalation is accompanied by a tightening of the muscles throughout the torso, including the abdominal muscles, the intercostal muscles in the chest and the muscles in the floor of the pelvis. At first, you will notice the abdominal muscles pressing the relaxed diaphragm up (and pushing the air out) with the chest in a relatively fixed position; then, you'll notice the chest being compressed inward and finally, toward the end of exhalation, you will notice the contraction of the pelvic diaphragm. This sequence of events will also take place if you breathe out normally, but creating resistance through pursed lips makes the muscular efforts much more obvious.

## A and P Breathing

This preliminary exercise to Agni Sara, called Akunchana Prasarana, or A and P breathing for short, involves active exhalations and relaxed inhalations. The literal meaning of the phrase is apt: "squeezing and releasing." Stand with the trunk pitched forward, the hands on the thighs just above the knees, the elbows extended, the feet about a foot and a half apart and the knees slightly bent. Much of the weight of the torso is placed on the front of the thighs. Breathe in and out a few times normally, and observe that the posture and the angle of the body pull the abdominal organs forward and create a mild tension against the abdominal wall. Notice that countering the tension produced by the force of gravity requires that a mild effort be made even at the beginning of exhalation and the greater the forward angle the greater the effect. To do A and P breathing, assume the same posture as in the trial run and press in slowly (squeezing) from all sides with the abdominal muscles as you exhale, all the while bolstering the effort with the chest. Your first impulse is to emphasize the upper abdomen. Try it several times, observing exactly where the various effects and sensations are felt. Notice that the effort in the upper abdomen is accompanied by a slight feeling of weakening in the lower abdomen. The lower region may not actually bulge out physically, but it feels as if it might. Now, try to exhale so that the upper abdomen, the lower abdomen and the sides are given equal emphasis, as though you are compressing a ball. Exhalation might take 6–7 seconds and inhalation 3–4. Inhalation is mostly passive (releasing) and manages itself naturally. Take 10–15 breaths in this manner. Much of inhalation is passive in A and P breathing because the chest springs open and the abdominal wall springs forward of its own accord. The strong emphasis on exhalation means that you are breathing in and out a tidal volume which is the combination of your normal tidal volume for an upright posture plus part of your expiratory reserve. Your revised tidal volume for A and P breathing might be about 900 ml for each breath rather than the textbook tidal volume of 500 ml. Along with this, your new expiratory reserve volume would become about 600 ml rather than 1,000 ml.

In any case, A and P breathing boosts your energy by increasing blood oxygen and decreasing blood carbon dioxide. It is a simple exercise but one that is both relaxing and invigorating.

## Agni Sara with Other Hatha Yoga Practices

If you are an advanced student, you can use Agni Sara (or A and P breathing) to intensify the hatha yoga postures in which you are comfortable. You will have to breathe faster than usual, of course, because the postures will increase your need for oxygen and carbon dioxide exchange. You will also have to modify the patterns of exhalation according to the demands of the posture. For example, in a deep standing forward bend you can both see and feel what is happening, but a standing backbend or spinal twist permits little obvious movement in the abdomen. That's fine. Either way, it's the attempt to press in from below that generates the surge of energy. And for all standing postures in which you are emphasizing an empowered thoracic inhalation, you can not only increase your inspiratory reserve volume by trying to inhale more deeply, you can use Agni Sara to exhale most or all of your expiratory reserve volume, thus inhaling and exhaling your vital capacity (the volume of which is specific to the particular posture) with every breath. After you have worked successfully with Agni Sara, bellows breathing and Kapalabhati for some time, you can experiment with an Agni Sara type of movement during the exhalation phases of the bellows breath and Kapalabhati.

Exhalation will produce an upward-moving wave of contraction—a pushing in and up sensation, rather than a mass contraction of the abdominal muscles. You can feel this if you span your hand across your abdomen with the middle finger on the navel, the thumb and index fingers above and the ring finger and little finger below. You will feel the little finger on the lower abdomen moving inward during exhalation, and little or no movement where the thumb is located on the upper abdomen. Using this technique for the bellows and Kapalabhati creates a mild scooping-up sensation. It requires more control than the standard techniques for bellows and Kapalabhati, so you will need to slow down—perhaps to as few as 60 breaths per minute. You will never be able to do it as fast as the standard technique, but it is still a powerful abdomino-pelvic exercise and is excellent for training the abdominal muscles for more advanced practices. Let's consider few more abdominal exercises for strong core strength.

## Abdomino-Pelvic Exercises

Yoga is concerned first and foremost with the inner life and abdomino-pelvic exercises are no exception. On the most obvious level, yoga postures strengthen the abdominal region and protect the back. But when you do them you also come alive with energy that can be felt from head to toe.

A sure way to develop what yogis call inner strength is to tone the abdominal region. If energy in arms and shoulder is weak, a strong abdomen can give you an extra edge, but if the abdomen is weak even the strongest arms and shoulder are likely to fail you.

Leg lifts, sit-ups, the sitting boat posture, and the peacock all create these effects through manipulating the limbs and torso in a gravitational field while you are using the abdominal region as a fulcrum for your efforts. The harder you work the more energizing the exercise. These seemingly diverse exercises not only strengthen the torso but also stimulate abdominal energy by using the abdomen as a fulcrum for manipulating large segments of the body in relation to one another in the field of gravity.

We have 4 pairs of abdominal muscles. Three of these form layers that encircle the abdomen and the fourth is a pair of longitudinal bands.

The external abdominal oblique layer runs diagonally from above downward in the same direction as the external intercostal muscles. If you place your hands in the pockets of a short jacket with your fingers extended, the fingers will point in the direction of external abdominal oblique muscle fibers.

The internal abdominal oblique layer is in the middle. Its fibers also run diagonally but in the opposite direction.

The innermost third layer, the transverse abdominis, runs horizontally around the abdominal wall from back to front. These three layers together act as a unit, helping to support the upper body and contributing to bending, twisting and turning in a logical fashion. They are also necessary for coughing, sneezing, laughing and various yoga breathing exercises.

The fourth pair of abdominal muscles, the rectus abdominis muscle (rectus means straight) runs vertically on either side of the midline between the pubic bone and the sternum. The rectus abdominis muscles are the prime movers (agonists) for flexion of the spine in crunches, while the hip flexors serve as synergists for bracing the pelvis and lumbar region.

Abdomino-pelvic exercises in detail:

1. Supine leg lifts.

    Start with the thighs adducted, the knees extended and the feet also extended, which means toes pointed away from you. The hands should be alongside the thighs, palms down. Now, slowly raise one foot as high as possible and then slowly lower it back to the floor. Repeat on the other side. Keep breathing and repeat several times.

    a. The bicycle and other variations:

    To prepare for more difficult yoga postures, after double leg-lift flex both knees and draw them towards the chest. Then, bicycle your feet around and around. Intensify even more by straightening the knees and pressing the feet towards the ceiling. You can also create scissoring motion, with the feet meeting midway or near the highest position.

    When you do variations that are more demanding than the simple bicycling motion, you will find that your abdominal muscles tighten, increasing intra-abdominal pressure and pressing the lower back against the floor in co-operation with the respiratory diaphragm.

    b. The fire exercise:

    When you become comfortable doing leg-lifts, bicycling and their variations for 5–10 minutes, then you can try the fire exercise. Fire exercise has been so named for its energizing effect on the body as a whole. To get into the position, sit on the floor, lean back, support yourself on the forearms and place the hands under the hips. Keeping the feet together, extend the toes, feet and knees and draw the head forward while keeping the back rounded. Exhale, and at the same time, slowly lift the feet as high as possible, drawing the extended knees toward the head. Slowly, come back down. Come up and down as many times as you can without strain, inhaling as required and always breathing evenly. If coming all the way up and down is difficult, simply tighten the muscle, lift the feet an inch or so, and hold in that position isometrically. A few days later, you will have enough strength to do the full exercise.

    c. Super fish leg-lift:

2. Yoga sit-ups.

3. Sitting boat posture.

4. Peacock posture.

Therapeutic benefits of abdomino-pelvic exercises:

Developing strength, increasing flexibility and improving aerobic capacity is important for physical conditioning. Yogis insist that these are the benefits of leg lifts, the peacock, Agni Sara, Uddiyana Bandha and Nauli. If we analyze, keeping in mind the anatomy and physiology of human body, these exercises

- Increase blood oxygen level and decrease blood carbon dioxide
- Stimulate adrenaline glands to release adrenaline and steroids
- Stimulate the release of glucagon from the islets of Langerhans in the pancreas
- Cause the liver to release extra glucose into the general circulation reducing appetite.

To experience these benefits, carry out a small experiment. The next time you feel hungry, instead of eating, practice 20 leg lifts and 10 minutes of Agni Sara. Immediately, you start to feel great and energetic even without eating. Amazing, but true. This is how yogis used to be fit and fine with little food consumption.

Lastly, I would like to mention that it may take many months to acquire the control and stamina necessary to perform this group of exercises, especially Agni Sara, correctly. Do not become discouraged. Your efforts will be rewarded with excellent health.

## Uddiyana Bandha, the Abdominal Lift

Mula Bandha seals the anatomical perineum, and Agni Sara teaches us special skills for using the abdominal muscles. When you have become proficient in both, you are ready to learn the second great lock in hatha yoga: Uddiyana Bandha or the abdominal lift.

To do it, you must exhale, hold your breath out (as it's said in yoga) and create a vacuum in your chest that sucks your diaphragm and abdominal organs to a higher than usual position in the torso. This can happen only if the body is sealed above and below—above at the glottis and below at the perineum. Without these seals air would be drawn into the larynx and lungs above, and into the eliminatory and reproductive organs below. You hold the root lock reflex and without having to think about it, the glottis has to be held shut voluntarily.

The best time to practice the abdominal lift is early in the morning, certainly before breakfast and ideally after having evacuated the bowels. The same contraindications apply as in Agni Sara (see the end of this chapter).

To begin, stand with your knees slightly bent and your hands braced against the thighs. As with Agni Sara, this stance lowers the abdominal organs downward and forward. Exhale to your maximum. Notice that you do this by pressing in first with the abdomen and then with the chest. Then, do mock inhalations with the chest, closing the glottis to restrain air from entering the lungs and at the same time, relax the abdomen. You should feel the chest lift. Holding the glottis closed for a few seconds, try harder to inhale, keeping the abdomen relaxed. The upper abdomen will form a deep concavity that extends up and underneath the rib cage. This is Uddiyana Bandha.

If you get confused about how to prevent air from entering the lungs, forget about the abdominal lift for a week or so and simply practice trying to inhale after full exhalations while you are blocking your mouth and nose with your hands.

Uddiyana Bandha: A maximum exhalation is followed by a mock inhalation with locked glottis and chin lock in combination with relaxed abdominal muscles.

To make holding the glottis shut feel more natural and comfortable, a third lock, Jalandhara Bandha (the chin lock), can be established by flexing the head forward so the chin is tucked into the suprasternal notch, the little concavity above the sternum at the pit of the throat. It is possible to do the abdominal lift without the chin lock, but its addition will make the closure of the glottis feel more secure, and many teachers consider it absolutely necessary. Fixing the eyes in a downward position also complements both Uddiyana Bandha and Jalandhara Bandha. Try looking up as you try them and you'll quickly sense the efficacy of looking down. Come out of Uddiyana Bandha in 2 stages. First, while still holding the glottis shut, ease the vacuum in the chest by relaxing the external intercostal muscles, which will lower the dome of the diaphragm and the abdominal organs to a lower position in the trunk. Then, as soon as the abdominal wall is eased forward, press inward strongly with the chest and abdomen until the pressure above and below the glottis is equalized. You have to compress inward just as forcefully as when you first exhaled for Uddiyana Bandha; if you don't, air will rush in with a gasp when you open the glottis. As soon as the pressure is equalized, open the glottis and breathe in gently.

Where does the vacuum come from?

In Uddiyana Bandha we are trying to inhale without inhaling, and this makes the thoracic cage larger, expanding it from side to side and from front to back. Since no air is allowed in, the air pressure inside the chest has to decrease, which, in turn, creates enough of a vacuum to pull the diaphragm up (provided it is relaxed) in proportion to the expansion of the rib cage. Coming down from Uddiyana Bandha, the side-to side and front-to-back expansions of the chest are first relaxed and then compressed back into their starting positions of full exhalation, and the dome of the diaphragm and abdominal organs move inferiorly.

Uddiyana Bandha is the only practice in hatha yoga that frankly stretches the respiratory diaphragm. It's true that you get a mild stretch of the diaphragm when you exhale as much as possible in Agni Sara and in the exhalation stage of Uddiyana Bandha, both of which push the dome of the diaphragm (from below) to the highest possible position the abdominal muscles can accomplish. But Uddiyana Bandha goes beyond this, because the vacuum in the chest that is superimposed on full exhalation pulls the diaphragm (from above) to an even higher position. We can surmise that regular practice of Uddiyana Bandha will stretch and, in time, lengthen the diaphragm's muscle and connective tissue fibers, as well as keep the zone of apposition between the diaphragm and the chest wall healthy and slippery. You will be able to exhale more completely as you gradually lengthen the muscle fibers, and you will be able to breathe more comfortably and efficiently as you increase the diaphragm's mobility.

## Problems

Many people, including yoga teachers, surprisingly, seem to have a great deal of difficulty learning Uddiyana Bandha. It is partly a matter of poor body awareness in the torso but the most constant factor is simply your history. Many youngsters grow up doing the abdominal lift in play, often combining it with other manipulations such as rolling the rectus abdominis muscles from side to side or up and down. Among a typical group of children, almost half will be able to do Uddiyana Bandha after only a few seconds of instruction and demonstration, and in a beginning hatha class for adults, those who did Uddiyana Bandha in play as children will usually be able to learn the yoga version immediately.

If you're having trouble, you are doing one of three things wrong.

1. You may not be exhaling enough at the start. The less you exhale, the less convincing the lift will be. You have to exhale the entire expiratory reserve volume—only the residual volume of air should remain in the lungs.

2. You may be letting in a little air on your mock inhalation. You have to try to inhale without doing so. That is the whole point of locking the airway at the glottis.

3. You are not relaxing the abdomen during the mock inhalation. You must learn to distinguish between pressing in with the abdominal muscles, which we want only for the preliminary exhalation, and allowing the abdominal wall to be pulled in passively by the vacuum in the chest. Many students hold their abdominal muscles rigidly or even try to keep pushing in with them during the lifting phase of the practice, and this prevents the abdominal organs and abdominal wall from being sucked in and up. It is also common for students to relax their abdominal muscles momentarily but then get mixed up and try to assist the inward movement with an active contraction. It won't work. You have to relax the abdominal muscles totally and keep them relaxed to do this exercise.

## Another Modified Cat Stretch

If you consistently have trouble relaxing the abdominal muscles for Uddiyana Bandha in a standing position, try it in a cat stretch, similar to the one we used for exploring Mula Bandha, but more relaxed. Rest on the knees and forearms and lower the forehead down against the crossed hands. Press the shoulders toward the floor and increase the lumbar arch as much as possible. This position pitches the abdominal and pelvic organs forward and toward the chest. Now, all you have to do is exhale as much as possible (which rounds your back posteriorly) and hold your breath at the glottis. Now, relax, allowing the lower back to arch forward again, and notice that in this position it is unnatural to hold the abdominal muscles firmly. Uddiyana Bandha comes effortlessly as your chest cooperates with gravity in pulling the abdominal organs to a higher position in your torso. Finally, continuing to hold your breath and keeping the abdomen relaxed, slowly lift your head and shoulders. Come up on your hands, walk them toward your knees and onto your thighs ever so delicately, and carefully come into an upright kneeling position without tightening the abdomen. If you are successful, you will be doing Uddiyana Bandha.

## Fire Dhauti

Here is a simple exercise that some texts call Agni Sara and others refer to as Fire Dhauti.

Come into Uddiyana Bandha (standing) and continuing to hold your breath, alternately lower and then lift the abdominal organs by decreasing and increasing the size of the chest cage with the intercostal muscles. Each time the abdominal organs are lowered, the abdominal wall is pushed out, and each time the abdominal organs are lifted into the typical Uddiyana Bandha position, the abdominal wall is pulled in. It's a pumping action, and it is sometimes done fast, up to 2 times per second, but more frequently it is done about once per second. When doing Fire Dhauti, keep in mind that you see and feel most of the action in the belly, but that control of the maneuver depends on the chest as well as holding your breath after a full exhalation. The abdominal muscles themselves remain passive: they are pulled up passively by Uddiyana Bandha, and they are pressed back out by gravity and by the action of the chest. You keep holding the breath at the glottis, but the vacuum in the chest is diminished and even converted momentarily into a positive pressure as the diaphragm and abdominal organs are pressed inferiorly. You can do the pumping action, of course, only for the length of time that you can hold your breath. This practice is an excellent training exercise for those who are having trouble releasing the abdominal muscles in Uddiyana Bandha, because its vigorous up and down motion has the effect of freeing you from holding the abdominal muscles rigidly.

## Nauli

Nauli, which means "churning," is one of the most rewarding abdominopelvic practices.

To do it you must first do Uddiyana Bandha and then contract the rectus abdominis muscle, first on one side and then the other, creating a wavelike, side-to-side motion in the abdomen. The other abdominal muscles remain relaxed, leaving concavities lateral to the rectus abdominis on each side. To learn the exercise, most people first learn to isolate both rectus abdominis muscles at the same time after having established Uddiyana Bandha. Then, still holding Uddiyana Bandha, they learn to contract each rectus abdominis muscle individually, and finally they learn to coordinate the side-to-side motion for the final practice.

## Contraindications of These Kriyas
### 1. High Blood Pressure

If you have high blood pressure, even the mildest of abdomino-pelvic exercises should be approached gingerly. Even if you are on medication that successfully lowers your blood pressure, all intense abdomino-pelvic exercises should be avoided. Holding your breath at the glottis after inhalation is always contraindicated. Holding your breath after exhalation, as in Uddiyana Bandha, is less dangerous but also inadvisable because we would expect it to quickly increase venous return, that is, the flow of blood back to the heart.

### 2. Ulcers

Intense abdomino-pelvic practices are all contraindicated for anyone with stomach and duodenal ulcers except in the case of practices recommended by a holistic physician who is willing to advise you.

### 3. Hiatal Hernia

The esophagus passes through the respiratory diaphragm, through the esophageal hiatus and, under certain conditions, the upper part of the stomach may herniate through this region of the diaphragm into the thoracic cavity. This is called hiatal hernia. If you have occasional discomfort in that region after eating or if you have acute discomfort just under the left side of the rib cage while trying the Peacock, Uddiyana Bandha, or vigorous versions of the cobra, it may be that the differential between intra-abdominal pressure (which is higher) and intra-thoracic pressure (which is lower) is causing the problem. It is important to seek medical counsel from someone who is conversant with hatha yoga before continuing with any posture or exercise that causes such symptoms.

## 4. Inguinal Hernia

The inguinal canal, through which the testis passes around the time of birth on its way to the scrotum, is another region of weakness in which abdominal organs or, more commonly, a little fatty tissue, usually from the greater omentum can herniate out of the abdominal cavity. This condition—an inguinal hernia—can also occur in women, although it is less common than in men. If a little out-pouching of soft tissue appears on one or both sides of the groin when you are upright and if that out-pouching disappears back into the abdominal cavity when you are lying down, it is almost certainly an inguinal hernia. Such hernias will become more pronounced in any standing posture and in exercises such as the Peacock that increase intra-abdominal pressure. Bicycling, walking, running and sun salutations also commonly make inguinal hernias more prominent. But they are unpredictable: they can get worse quickly or remain about the same for months or years. If the condition is not repaired surgically, a support (truss) that presses against the hernia from the outside may be effective in keeping the contents of the abdomen out of the inguinal canal, but in the absence of such a device, strenuous upright postures and the Peacock should be avoided.

## 5. Menstruation and Pregnancy

No exercise involving breath retention should be practiced during menstruation or pregnancy, but the regular and enthusiastic practice of abdomino-pelvic exercises appears to be helpful in preventing premenstrual symptoms and cramping. During pregnancy, most practices in hatha yoga are contra-indicated, especially those that increase intra-abdominal pressure but also those few that decrease it, such as Uddiyana Bandha. Ashwini Mudra and Mula Bandha are fine and are even recommended during pregnancy, but Agni Sara is contraindicated because of its intensity. One caution for expert hatha yogis who have just given birth: the fascia that connects the 2 rectus abdominis muscles in the midline may have become weakened by pregnancy and childbirth, and women who were able to do the Peacock easily before having children are sometimes unable to do so afterwards because the rectus abdominis muscles are now pulled uncomfortably apart in the effort to come into the posture.

# Benefits

Everyone knows that developing strength, improving aerobic capacity and increasing flexibility is important for physical conditioning. The question of how to accomplish these goals is less certain, but yogis insist that these are the benefits of leg lifts, the Peacock, Agni Sara, Uddiyana Bandha and Nauli. Why that happens is still something of a mystery, but we can call on our experience to make some reasonable guesses. If you are hungry and tired, but feel great after doing 20 leg lifts and 10 minutes of Agni Sara instead of eating and taking a nap, something obviously worked—and anyone who has a little knowledge of anatomy and physiology can make intelligent guesses about what, where, and how. You increased your blood oxygen and decreased your blood carbon dioxide; you stimulated the adrenal glands to release epinephrine (adrenaline) and steroids; you stimulated the release of glucagon from the islets of Langerhans in the pancreas and your liver released extra glucose into the general circulation, cutting your appetite and preparing you for getting on with your day. We can also look at the physiology of any specific practice and comment on events that are certain to result. For example, we can note that any activity that increases intra-abdominal pressure while the airway is being kept open will force blood more efficiently than usual from the venous system in the abdominal region up into the chest. Quantities can be debated, measurements taken and opinions stated on how and why that might be beneficial, but there can be no argument about the reality of the effects.

"It may take many months to acquire the control and stamina necessary to perform this exercise (agni sara) correctly. Do not become discouraged. Your efforts will be rewarded with excellent health."

## Drishti

Now let's understand the Drishti or focal point. The fifth limb of yoga is Pratyahara, that is, sense withdrawal.

According to *Yoga Yajnavalkya*, which contains the yoga teachings of the sage Yajnavalkya, "One must endeavor to retain all the prana through the mind, in the navel, the tip of the nose and the big toes." Focusing at the tip of the nose is the means to gain mastery over prana. By focusing on the navel all diseases are removed. The body attains lightness by focusing on the big toes. According to A G Mohan, a student of T Krishnamacharya and translator of the *Yoga Yajnavalkya*, the aim of yoga is to concentrate the prana in the body, whereas it is usually scattered. A scattered prana will correspond to a scattered state of mind.

The Upanishads explain that the senses deliver the fuel for the mind in the form of sense objects. The mind then develops desires, which are the source of suffering.

The concept of yoga, on the other hand, holds that we are always in the original and pristine state of bliss, which is consciousness. This original state is formless, however, and since the mind has a tendency to attach itself to whatever comes along next, we forget our true nature. Sense withdrawal means to accept the fact that external stimuli can never truly fulfill us. Once that is accepted, we are free to realize that what we were desperately looking for outside was present inside all along. The Upanishads explain further that, as a fire dies down when the fuel is withheld, so the mind will return to its source when the fuel of the sense is withheld. This method can be brought about through sense withdrawal (Pratyahara).

The withdrawal of the audio sense is brought about by listening to one's own breath rather than to external sounds. The withdrawal or turning in of the visual sense is practiced through drishti, the attachment of one's gaze on various focal points. There are nine places to look, called nava drishtis:

1. Nasagra: the space just beyond the tip of the nose. This is used most often and is the primary drishti in the sitting postures.
2. Ajña chakra: the space between the eyebrows (third eye) (for example, the Purvottanasana/Intense East Stretch).

3. Nabi chakra: navel center (for example, Adho Mukha Svanasana/Downward-Facing Dog).

4. Hastagra: hand (for example, Trikonasana/Triangle).

5. Padhayoragrai: toes (for example, Savangasana/Shoulder Stand).

6. Parshva: far to the right (for example, Supta Padangusthasana/Reclining Big Toe posture).

7. Parshva: far to the left (for example, Marichyasana C/Marchi's posture).

8. Angushtha madya: thumbs (beginning of Suryanamaskara/Sun Salutation).

9. Úrdhva drishti or antara drishti: up to the sky (Virabhadrasana A/Warrior).

By doing this, one prevents oneself from looking around, which would make the mind reach outwards. Following drishti, the practice becomes deeply internal and meditative.

Drishti is also a practice of concentration (Dharana), the sixth limb of Patanjali's limbs of yoga. If we practice in a distracted way, we may find ourselves listening to the birds outside and gazing around the room. To perform all of the prescribed actions —Bandha, Ujjayi, Drishti—and find the proper alignment, the mind needs to be fully concentrated; otherwise, one of the elements will miss out. In this way, the practice provides us with constant feedback about whether we are in Dharana. In time, Dharana will lead to meditation (Dhyana).

In astanga vinyasa method, drishti is one of the vital techniques to draw the prana inwards. Anyone who has practiced in front of the mirror may have noticed how looking into it draws awareness away from the core towards the surface. This is exactly what happens to the flow of prana, which follows awareness. Practicing in front of the mirror might be helpful from time to time to check one's alignment if no teacher is present, but it is preferable to develop a proprioceptive awareness, one that does not depend on visual clues. This type of awareness draws Prana inwards, which corresponds to what the Upanishads call dissolving the mind into heart. The permanent establishing of prana in the core of the body leads to Samadhi or liberation.

# Vinyasa

Vinyasa yoga is a system of yoga specifically designed for householders. The difference between a householder and (Grihasta) and an enunciate (Sanyasi) is that the latter has no social duties and can therefore devote 10 or more hours per day to practice. In fact, if individual techniques pertaining to all 8 limbs were practiced daily, one would easily spend more than 10 hours practicing. For example, asana practice for 2 hours, pranayama for 2 hours, mudra and japa each for 1 hour, reading of scripture for 1 hour, chanting for 1 hour, reflection and contemplation for 1 hour and meditation for 1 hour.

A householder, meaning someone who has a family and a job or a business to attend to, can never spend so much time on practice.

Thus, to work for householders, yoga practice would have to be compressed into 2 hours and still retain its benefits. With this in mind, Rishi Vamana created vinyasa yoga. He arranged the practice in sequences, such that the postures were potentizing their effects, and combined them with mudra, pranayama and meditation so that a 10-hour practice could be effectively compressed into 2 hours.

One of vinyasa yoga's outstanding features is that postures are not held for a long time. The core idea is to shift emphasis from posture to breath and therefore to realize that postures, like all forms are impermanent. So, it is necessary to organize the practice in such a way that nothing impermanent is held on to. Vinyasa yoga is a meditation on impermanence. The only thing permanent in practice is the constant focus on the breath.

According to the *Brahma Sutra*, "Ata eva pranah," the breath verily is Brahman. The breath is here identified as a metaphor for Brahman (meaning deep reality, infinite consciousness). Through vinyasa, the postures are linked to form a mala. A mala is commonly used to count mantras during meditation. In vinyasa yoga, every asana becomes a bead on this mala of yoga postures. In this way, the practice becomes a movement meditation.

Vinyasa yoga practice produces heat, which is needed to burn toxins, not only physical toxins but also the toxin of ignorance and delusion. The full vinyasa practice, which entails coming back to standing between postures, has a flushing effect through constant forward bending. It is recommended in case of strong, persistent toxicity and for recuperation after disease. The half vinyasa practice, in which one jumps between performance of the right and left side sitting postures, is designed to create a balance between strength and flexibility and to increase heat.

If asana alone is practiced, it might lead to excess flexibility, which can destabilize the body. The proper position of the bones in the body, the spine, is remembered by sustaining a certain core tension in the muscles. If the tension is insufficient, frequent visits to an osteopath may become necessary. This possibility is avoided in vinyasa yoga by jumping back between sides, which give us the strength to support the flexibility gained in the practice. This concept is very important to understand. Flexibility that cannot be supported by strength should not be aimed for.

Patanjali, in *Yoga Sutra* II.48, quotes, "Thus one is un assailed by the pair of opposites." For this reason, one needs to place the same importance on vinyasa as on asana. The underlying principle here is that of simultaneous expansion into opposing directions. Whenever we expand into one direction, we at the same time need to counteract that by expanding into the opposite direction. In this way, we are not caught into extremes of body and mind.

## Applied anatomy of vinyasa flow

Vinyasa combines poses to flow one into another in sequence. Postures from the sun salutations form the foundation repeated in successive rounds. Individual poses are then inserted into this foundation to create diversity within the flow. These asanas become the centerpiece of each round of vinyasa.

The flow sequence encircles the centerpiece pose and is the "home base" to which we return. Central to this practice is the coupling of breath and movement. Vinyasa affects the body on many levels.

- It is an aerobic style of yoga that generates heat from muscle metabolism. Surface blood vessels then dilate to release this heat. This combines with sweating to maintain normal body temperature, producing a healthy glow to the skin and releasing toxins. Because you can sweat a great deal during practice, be sure to drink plenty of water (at room temperature, not cold) to maintain hydration.

- The repetitive nature of vinyasa takes the joints through an increasingly greater range of motion, improving the circulation of synovial fluid and bringing nutrients to the articular cartilage. Working the muscles increases their metabolic rate, causing a slight rise in body temperature, which improves pliability in the ligaments and tendons.

- Alternately contracting and stretching the muscles during vinyasa augments blood flow by compressing and expanding the veins. Cardiac output also increases.

- Rhythmic contraction and relaxation of the diaphragm during breathing massages the abdominal organs and improves their function. Ujjayi breathing also produces a resonant sound that echoes throughout the physical body, connecting it to universal vibrational energies. Allow your breath to be the background soundtrack for your practice, like waves rolling onto a beach covered with smooth round stones. Breathing in this manner will eventually produce a self-sustaining rhythmic vibration. Combining breath and muscle work creates a symphony of movement and a resonance that will carry over into your daily life.

Vinyasa flow can be used to warm the body for other types of practice or can embody the practice itself. Think of vinyasa flow as a multilayered system that combines breath work, muscle activation and rhythmic movement. Transition smoothly from one pose to the next, and progressively refine each successive round.

Begin by warming up the muscles that are the prime movers of the major joints. These are the muscles that create the general form of the pose. For example, in Downward-Facing Dog, begin by engaging the quadriceps to straighten the knees and the triceps to extend the elbows. This stretches antagonist muscles, including the hamstrings and biceps. Consciously contracting the prime movers of the joints has the additional physiological effect of relaxing their antagonist muscles through reciprocal inhibition. As your practice session progresses, incorporate other muscles to reinforce the poses.

# Chapter 3

# ASANA KINESIOLOGY

Many students want to know if what they are feeling is correct. This is an excellent question and the answer varies.

In the Structural Yoga approach to Classical Yoga, the student is directed to hold the pose so that attention is upon the specific sites feeling the sensations of stretch and strength. The beginner often reports feeling the poses all over. This is normally a sign that sensitivity has not been attained. When there is too much sensation, the student may be overwhelmed and thus unable to determine where or what is being felt.

It takes time to understand anatomy and yet remain detached enough from that intellectual knowledge to gain somatic knowledge of the feeling in your mind/body. Many regular students cannot distinguish the feeling of stretch from those of strengthening. While this may seem to be an astonishing statement, it is quite true. Even yoga students of many years fail to think clearly about their experience of practice, especially in intricate asanas where the body is doing several joint motions simultaneously. For instance, in simple cross-legged sitting, it is not easy to determine what one feels in the musculature. The knees are flexed, the hips are flexed, and they are externally rotated. This combination of joint motions requires discrimination to perceive kinesthetically and to understand intellectually what is occurring in the musculature. With anatomical mindfulness and detachment as core to their training, students will be able to give details on the specific areas reacting to a posture.

A beautiful practice of yogasana is a work of art or, more accurately, it is a combination of a work of art and a work of diligent persistent effort guided by discrimination. As you continue to practice yogasanas, you may find yourself wondering if you are doing poses properly or feeling the poses in the right places. This is a good question to continue to ask yourself.

## Where Should I Feel the Pose?

For students on the beginning level, there is a right and wrong way to do yoga poses. There is a correct appearance and correct feel for postures. The right way will alleviate the sources of your stress and physical tension. The right way is when the pain feels good. Where you feel the poses will vary according to your postural imbalances, your strength and your flexibility. The table provided on the kinesiology of yoga asanas later in this chapter illustrates the 24 poses of the Structural Yoga Therapy routine and the ideal muscles that will be strengthened and stretched.

This summary is misleading, however, unless you remember your specific postural imbalances. Muscles will not stretch or strengthen normally when there are postural imbalances. The shape of your bones may be different from that shown in pictures in anatomy atlases. These 2 factors will give your body feelings in places different from that of other students.

I encourage students in my classes to tell me where they feel the poses for two reasons. First, I want them to be practicing self-observation as much as possible. By focusing your attention on yourself, you are more inclined to self-adjust and lessen your tension. Second, I want to protect them from hurting themselves or working in detrimental ways. Since I know anatomy and yoga better than most of my students, I know where the safe and unsafe places are in every posture.

For students who practice irregularly, but are not beginners, most of these considerations are also valid. For them, however, additional concern is needed to provide motivation for establishing regularity. The need is there to keep the practice at a level of intensity that is fresh, insightful and stimulating, yet not overly aggressive.

For students on the committed level, yoga is a personal practice aimed at getting to know yourself. For them, there really is no wrong way to do poses. Regular reading of the guidelines given in Patanjali's *Yoga Sutras* will definitely deepen the experiences available from yoga practice.

The table on the kinesiology of yoga asanas (later in this chapter) summarizes ideal places to focus your intention to strengthen and stretch. The movements and muscles cited are optimal for receiving the benefits of the poses. Be gentle and do not demand that your body feel the effects as cited. Persist, nonetheless, at consistently guiding yourself to find these places of your anatomy while in the yogasanas.

The table is based upon practices as described in this book and asanas from the text of BKS Iyengar in his *Light on Yoga*. As his method is well accepted for its precision of anatomical placement, it is the most readily usable method of Hatha Yoga for this study. The table lists the poses to strengthen and stretch the muscles indicated in the middle column. Three poses are given for each purpose, listed in the order of their effectiveness at working the complete combinations of actions of the muscle cited.

## Gravity—an Additional Factor in Asana Kinesiology

The effects of gravity cannot be underemphasized. The same pose done in different body placements provides an extremely different benefit to the musculoskeletal system. An astute student will notice in the Structural Yoga Therapy series that there are several postures in which the body is at a right angle (90 degrees) of hip flexion. These include Downward-Facing Dog, Upward Stretched Legs, Supported Shoulder Stand, Stick and the Complete Boat.

To this, one could add the preliminary motion of the Half-Forward Bend, and the more advanced Plow Pose (Halasana). In each instance, there is a contraction of the hip flexors (rectus femoris, psoas, tensor fascia lata and sartorius) and a stretch of the hip extensors (hamstrings and gluteus maximus). In each, the relationship of the body to gravity is changed, so the kinesiological effects are different. For instance, to compare the effects on the hamstrings in these poses, the pull is mildest in the Complete Boat and Inverted Action poses and somewhat greater in Stick Pose. Yet, most students do not feel these effects unless their hamstrings are extremely short. The effectiveness of stretching the hamstrings is more pronounced in Half-Forward Bend and a full stretch is usually experienced in Downward-Facing Dog Pose.

Similarly, if we compare these poses for their effectiveness in strengthening the hip flexors, the effect is mild in the Inverted Action Pose, stronger in the Stick Pose and most challenging in the Downward-Facing Dog and Complete Boat poses. By taking these factors into consideration, we can grade the level of difficulty more precisely when composing your personalized Structural Yoga Therapy program.

## Designing Your Personal Program

By summarizing the muscles, you need to strengthen and muscles you need to stretch, you have created a thorough evaluation. The next step will be to find yoga poses that stretch and strengthen the specific muscles you want to change.

The first line of the table below shows the muscles strengthened and the second line the poses that stretch the muscle. The poses on each line are ranked for three levels of intensity. The first pose cited will produce a mild effect, the second a moderate effect. The third pose presents the strongest challenge to the muscle. From this, you can find the appropriate asana to practice for a personalized program. To create the most effective practice, you will need to sequence the program properly.

### *The Kinesiology of Yoga Asanas*

| Body Region | Muscles Affected | Yoga Poses to Strengthen and Stretch |
|---|---|---|
| Neck | Sternocleidomastoid Flexion, Lateral Rotation | Strengthen: Spinal Twist, Extended Triangle, Camel<br><br>Stretch: Twisting poses |
| | Upper Trapezius Extension | Stretch: Bridge, Shoulder Stand, Plow |
| Shoulder | Middle Deltoid/Supraspinatus Abduction to 90 degrees | Strengthen: Extended Triangle, Warrior II, Side Body Support<br><br>Stretch: Seated Spinal Twist, Face of Light, Eagle |
| | Anterior Deltoid/Coracobrachialis Flexion to 90 degrees, Internal Rotation | Strengthen: Balancing Tree, Downward-Facing Dog, Eagle<br><br>Stretch: Stick, Camel, Plow |

| Body Region | Muscles Affected | Yoga Poses to Strengthen and Stretch |
|---|---|---|
|  | Posterior Deltoid<br><br>Extension, External Rotation | Strengthen: Cobra, Bow, Supported Shoulder Stand<br><br>Stretch: Downward-Facing Dog, Face of Light, Reverse Namaste |
|  | Pectoralis Major Flexion, Adduction, Internal Rotation | Strengthen: Stick. Energy-Freeing Pose, Spinal Twist<br><br>Stretch: Cobra, Camel, Downward-Facing Dog |
|  | Teres Major<br><br>Extension, Adduction, Internal Rotation | Strengthen: Camel, Cobra, Plow |
|  | Teres Minor Adduction, External Rotation | Strengthen: Camel, Supported Shoulder Stand, Bow<br><br>Stretch: Downward-Facing Dog, Spinal Twist, Face of Light<br><br>Stretch: Cat, Spinal Twist, Face of Light |
|  | Triceps Brachii<br><br>Shoulder and Elbow Flexion<br><br>Supination of the Forearm | Strengthen: Cobra, Stick, Supported Shoulder Stand<br><br>Stretch: Reverse Namaste, Revolving Head-to-Knee, Face of Light |
|  | Latissimus Dorsi Extension, Adduction, Internal Rotation<br><br>Lateral Flexion and Rotation of Spine | Strengthen: Camel, Spinal Twist, Shoulder Stand<br><br>Stretch: Energy Freeing, Abdominal Twist, Westside Back stretch |
| Scapula | Middle and Lower Trapezius Adduction, Depression | Strengthen: Bridge, Camel, Cat Bows<br><br>Stretch: Cat (back up), Head-to-Knee, Westside Back Stretch |

*Cont'd...*

[95]

| Body Region | Muscles Affected | Yoga Poses to Strengthen and Stretch |
| --- | --- | --- |
| | Serratus Anterior Abduction, Elevation | Strengthen: Energy Freeing, Crow, Head-to-Knee Pose<br><br>Stretch: Cobra, Camel, Spinal Twist |
| | Rhomboids<br>Adduction, Elevation | Strengthen: Cobra, Camel, Reverse Namaste<br><br>Stretch: Cat (back down), Stick, Spinal Twist |
| Spine | Erector Spinae Extension, Lateral Flexion, Rotation | Strengthen: Cobra, Extended Triangle, Locust<br><br>Stretch: Extended Triangle, Side Angle Pose, Westside Back Stretch |
| | Rectus Abdominis Flexion; Lateral Flexion, Rotation, Pelvic Thrust | Strengthen: Upward Stretch Legs, Boat, Nauli<br><br>Stretch: Cobra, locust, Bow |
| | Abdominis Oblique Lateral Flexion, Rotation | Strengthen: Extended Triangle, Spinal Twist, Abdominal Twist<br><br>Stretch: Same poses on the opposite side of muscles |
| Hip | Psoas<br>Flexion, External Rotation | Strengthen: Energy Freeing, Stick, Westside Back Stretch<br><br>Stretch: Camel, Bow, Reclining Hero |
| | Gluteus Maximus Extension, External Rotation | Strengthen: Bridge, Camel, Locust<br><br>Stretch: Energy Freeing, Westside Back Stretch, Squat Pose |
| | Gluteus Medius Extension, Abduction, Internal and External Rotation | Strengthen: Balancing Tree, Extended Triangle, Locust<br><br>Stretch: Side of Hip Stretch, Spinal Twist, Head to Knee |

| Body Region | Muscles Affected | Yoga Poses to Strengthen and Stretch |
|---|---|---|
| | External Rotators Abduction, External Rotation | Strengthen: Balancing Tree, Head-to-Knee, Bound Angle<br>Stretch: Side of Hip Stretch, Eagle, Face of Light<br>Strengthen: Bridge, Locust, Camel Pose<br>Stretch: Side of Hip Stretch, Extended Triangle, Westside Back Stretch |
| | Hamstrings<br>Extension, Knee Flexion | Strengthen: Energy Freeing, Side Angle, Spread Leg Stretch<br>Stretch: Spinal Twist, Joint Freeing Series #7, Face of Light |
| | Tensor Fascia Lata Abduction, Flexion, Internal Rotation | Strengthen: Side of Hip Stretch, Warrior I, Bound Angle<br>Stretch: Camel, Bow, Runner's Stretch |
| | Sartorius<br>Flexion,<br>Abduction, External Rotation with Knee Flexion | Strengthen: Warrior II, Upward Stretched Legs, Boat<br>Stretch: Bridge, Runner's Stretch, Camel |
| | Rectus Femoris<br>Flexion of Hip, Knee Flexion | Strengthen: Cobra, Warrior I, Side of Hip Stretch<br>Stretch: Triangle, Bound Angle, Seated Angle Stretch |
| | Adductors<br>Adduction, Hip Flexion | Strengthen: Side of Hip Stretch, Bridge, Bow<br>Stretch: Head to Knee, Bound Angle, Seated Angle Stretch |
| | Gracilis<br>Adduction, Hip and Knee Flexion | |

*Cont'd...*

| **Body Region** | **Muscles Affected** | **Yoga Poses to Strengthen and Stretch** |
|---|---|---|
| Knee | Quadriceps Knee Extension | Strengthen: Warrior I and II, Squat<br><br>Stretch: Energy Freeing, Hero, Camel |
| | Gastrocnemius<br><br>Knee Flexion, Ankle Plantar Flexion | Strengthen: Mountain on toes, Eagle, Squat on toes<br><br>Stretch: Extended Triangle, Warrior I, Downward-Facing Dog |
| Ankle | Anterior Tibialis Dorsiflexion, Inversion | Strengthen: Extended Triangle, Downward-Facing Dog, Squat<br><br>Stretch: Stick, Hero, Fetal |
| | Posterior Tibialis Plantar Flexion, Inversion | Strengthen: Hero, Camel, Hero with Knees Lifted<br><br>Stretch: Warrior I, Downward-Facing Dog, Squat |
| | Soleus<br>Plantar Flexion | Strengthen and Stretch: Same as Posterior Tibialis |
| | Peroneous Longus and Brevis<br>Dorsiflexion, Eversion | Strengthen: Extended Triangle, Spread Leg Stretch with Toes Outward<br><br>Stretch: Lotus, Hero, Reclining Hero with Toes Inward |

# Where Shouldn't I Feel the Pose?

This is an important issue to keep in mind during any form of exercise. There are 2 areas of the body where one should never feel a reaction from any activity, and most certainly not as a result of a yoga pose. These areas are the inner knees and the sacroiliac joints. Neither of these areas is covered by muscles or contractile tissue. They possess only ligaments for stability. Since ligaments do not stretch, these areas are particularly vulnerable to pain from activities that place stress upon them. These 2 areas of the body lack muscles to provide stability and resilience.

The region of the inner knees lies between the kneecap (patella) and the tripod tendons that form the lower ends (insertion points) for three muscles—the gracilis (an adductor), sartorius (the longest muscle in the body, an external hip rotator) and the semi membranosis (the most medial hamstring). In addition, all three muscles flex the knee joint. In the inner knee space, there are only ligaments and cartilage to provide stability and mobility to the knee. The most familiar of these structures are the anterior cruciate ligament and the medial meniscus (cartilage). The knee does not allow the twisting or lateral movements that are commonly required of activities like skiing, tennis or golf. Some martial arts warm up with knee circles, which are potentially harmful to this region. In yoga poses, pay particular attention to bent-knee poses with hip rotation, such as cross-legged sitting, as in the Lotus position, or forward-bending poses like the Head-to-Knee Pose and its variations.

This area is vulnerable to postures in which the foot is planted and the knee is not aligned to the foot. This sometimes occurs during practice of the Warrior poses for students who do not keep a back leg firmly extended. Another pose in which the knee is vulnerable is sitting between the feet with the feet turned outward, an uncommon variation of the Hero Pose (Virasana).

The sacroiliac is located at the base of the spine, where the sacrum, composed of five fused vertebrae, joins the iliac pelvic bones on its left and right sides. In men, the joint is more stable as three sacral vertebrae join the iliac, while in women; only 2 connect to the iliac. They may be seen on some slender individuals as dimples above the buttocks. The sacroiliac joints should have a subtle mobility, but should never be stretched, as they possess only ligaments to maintain their integrity. Ligaments do not stretch. I have come across some long-term women yoga teachers who have chronic pain in this area, caused from stretching this joint. This often comes about during spinal twisting motions and extremes of forward-bending poses. These should be done so that the stretch is felt in the deep buttock or hip-joint area.

The sacral area is vulnerable to forward bends, especially seated poses done with the knees straight. This is the case in the Head-to-Knee Pose and the Westside Back Stretch Pose. If this area is felt, adjust the pose so that the stretch is felt in the middle or lower back or into the hamstring muscles. By following instructions carefully, there is no danger in yoga poses. Above all, you must learn to be sensitive to your body as the home of your inner teacher and allow your intuition to guide you. After all, yoga is a journey that can take you back home, so don't get sidetracked by the scenery along the way.

Another important feature to watch for during yogasanas is excessive mobility. If you know you have hyperextended knees or elbows, or in general are simply naturally flexible, be cautious of where you feel your poses. This is especially true when you are holding the poses for a long time and when you find yourself repeating the same postures for relieving your stress. Hypermobile joints tend to become overused. The surrounding muscle tissue will often lack muscle tone, firmness and stamina. A locked joint, while providing stability, lacks mobility and the ability to adapt to change. Personality and joints live in the same body/mind, so they may resemble each other.

When doing yoga poses with straight arms or legs, such as Warrior poses, standing forward bends, Downward-Facing Dog, Stick Pose and Spinal Twists, be cautious that you are not locked into position. Rather, keep the ability to change your flexibility every time you do these poses. See if you can focus your awareness on strongly contracting specific muscles within these poses. If you can, then chances are you are not locking your joints.

For standing poses, as a test of locked knees, I often encourage students to lift their toes and see if the posture remains the same or changes. If your knees are locked, you'll move. Locking the joints blocks the flow of mindfulness, making it unable for you to experience other parts of yourself. It's important to be able to move your awareness to any part of your body at will.

It is fascinating to note that advanced students report feeling the pose all over. This is because their mind/body has been refined from focusing on a gross physical body, to one of sensing energy and sensation (subtle emotion). In this case, the energy body of prana has been trained to flow evenly throughout the system, and the mind has been trained to witness these subtle emotions and energy patterns. Over time, the irregularities in each body have been worked through. The student becomes stable and peaceful in situations that formerly would have proved stressful.

Since most people have postural imbalances and resulting muscle imbalances, the places where the pose is felt will vary. By taking the time for a postural analysis, you will identify which muscles to stretch and which ones to strengthen to achieve better alignment. Next, referring to the table above, you can locate the poses to practice for your specific muscle stretching and strengthening needs. Studying anatomy will enable you to greatly amplify the efficiency of yoga asanas, which will, in turn, promote a balance between your muscles' capacity for strength and stability and for flexibility and openness.

The short-term benefit of attention to anatomy is a strengthening of areas of weakness and a stretching of specific areas of tightness. In this way, your body functions more efficiently. Less effort is required to perform your daily activities. In the long run, especially if you receive personal guidance from an experienced instructor, your posture will improve, the residual effects of injuries will diminish and your performance of athletic activities will be enhanced.

## Principles for Good Practice

There are several other elements that will enhance the benefits of your yoga practice. It is most important that you begin with and maintain throughout practice an open mind and receptivity, allowing the yoga to benefit you in any way. It is also very important that you let go of expectations. I say to new students, "Leave your expectations at the door with your shoes." We are all multidimensional beings. The experiences of yoga affect us on all levels of body, mind and spirit. The region of the body where the predominant effect is found or felt will also vary from day to day. So, even if you come to yoga to relieve your chronic backache, along the way you may become aware of your physically held emotions. The variety of inner work accompanying yoga is as unique as the students who come to it. While there is a right place to feel the pose for you as an individual, there is no right time or place for your emotional and mental issues to come into the light of awareness. As you practice these structural yoga asanas, you will discover that your body begins to change. The postural changes may not be apparent at first. You may find changes on the level of increased flexibility or in the ease of holding a pose, indicative of increased strength. Over time, these changes will affect your body segment alignment and, thus, your posture as a whole. Aligning ankles to knees, knees to hips, hips to shoulders, shoulders to head, in this order, will progressively stabilize your new posture. In practicing the postures, always correct your alignment from the lower joints to the upper.

## *The Base of Support*

One important concept of the inner work with structural yoga asanas is called the base of support. This refers to the idea that each segment of the body is supported from below. If the segment below is misaligned, the segment above will tend to become misaligned, unstable and uncomfortable. Hence, an awareness of discomfort is heightened, because the body pan below where you feel the stress is not providing support. While instability is felt in the segment that is out of alignment, the cause is often from its base of support being misaligned. In correcting postural misalignments, therefore, it is recommended that you work from the ground up. In standing postures, correct the ankles, then knees and so on, up to the neck. For instance, if there has been chronic neck pain, it is not recommended to put much effort into realigning the neck until much work has been placed into correcting the shoulders and upper back. In terms of aligning within an asana, do not correct for your neck until you have corrected misalignments from your ankles up to knees, to hips, to back, then to the neck. Often, when adjusting your body in this manner, the base of support is reestablished for each segment and this will alleviate discomfort in the more superior joints. Hence, your neck will adapt to the lower segments and become much more comfortable, without directly correcting its position. In all postures, the progression for correcting alignment is to start from the base of support, that is, from the ground and precede upward, one joint at a time. In so doing, the upper body will automatically align itself around a more stable, comfortable, aligned base of support. To get the most from your practice, it is important to keep in mind the overview of yoga. A common pitfall in practicing yoga is forgetting yoga principles to achieve competence in Hatha Yoga. To avoid this and stay on track, I suggest you read and reread the opening chapters of this book. I also highly recommend reading *The Crown of Life* by Kirpal Singh, a wonderful book that puts the entire range of human development into a yogic perspective.

## Sequence for Mastery

There is a progression I recommend in order to thoroughly learn the practices of Structural Yoga Therapy.

1. Learn the position from the "how to" portion of the instructions.
2. Study the major muscle and joint actions cited, so that you can develop clarity on the focal motions recommended for the posture.
3. Train yourself to follow the experiential sequence cited in the *Yoga Sutra* (II, 46), learning to become steady and comfortable in the posture and in the movements leading into and out of the posture. To deepen the practice, the next sutra recommends that yoga posture be perfected through "relaxation of effort, lessening the tendency for restlessness, and identification with the Infinite stream of life." This is, of course, a never-ending story, revealing the intention of yoga to be a method of attaining reintegration with our True Selves.

# Chapter 4

# PRANAYAMA
# (CONSCIOUS BREATHING)

## Definition of Prānāyāma

Prana is life force and cosmic energy and ayama is regulation and restraint. Prānāyāma is the art of breathing; it leads to control of the mind, resulting in emotional stability, concentration and meditative stage.

Prānāyāma bridges the mind, body and soul and serves as a vehicle to a journey of self-realization: a state of joy and happiness. The grossest manifestation of prana in the human body is the motion of the lungs. This motion acts like a flywheel that sets other forces of the body in motion.

The practice of prānāyāma is to control the motion of the lungs, by which the prana is controlled. When the subtle prana is controlled, all gross manifestation of prana in the physical body will slowly come under control. When we concentrate and consciously regulate breathing, we are able to generate and store a greater amount of prana and energy. A person who has abundant pranic energy radiates vitality and strength. This can be felt by all who come into contact with him or her.

In Patanjali's 195 Sanskrit sutra, he described Ashtanga as eight limbs yoga. The eight limbs are the yama, niyama, āsana, pranayama, pratyāhāra, dhāranā, dhyāna and samādhi. In the system of Ashtanga yoga, prānāyāma, the fourth limb, is practiced to make breath long, deep, subtle and meditative. Like other limbs it prepares practitioners to the state of samādhi.

Mechanically, prānāyāma consists of inhalation (puraka), exhalation (rechaka) and retention (kumbhaka). The subtle control of the three parts requires practice and dedication. It leads to longevity of life due to slower breath, according to BKS Iyengar.

## Preparation for Prānāyāma

Place yourself in a comfortable sitting pose, Padmasana (Lotus), Bhadrasana (Half Lotus), Swasticasana (Cross-Legged), Virasana (Hero Pose), sitting on a chair with feet flat on the floor and upper legs parallel to the floor or laying down on the floor (Savasana) with a straight back and tuck in the forefinger and middle finger of your right hand. Use the right thumb to control your right nostril and right ring finger and pinky finger to control your left nostril. Guruji explains the purpose of this hand mudra: when we practice prānāyāma, it has nothing to do with our inner soul (index finger) and our intellect (middle finger) so these 2 fingers are tucked away while we make a connection between our super soul (thumb) and body (ring finger) and mind (pinky finger).

# Pranayama Techniques

## *Breathe Awareness*

Take a comfortable position—sit, stand, lie down facing up or be in any posture and breathe slowly and consciously. Then, direct your attention to the following:

- Feel the rise and fall of the abdomen.
- Feel the rise and fall of the chest.
- Be aware of long, deep and subtle inhalations and exhalations.
- Be aware of cool air entering the nostrils, throat and lungs and warm air exiting the lungs, throat and nostrils.
- Be aware of rising energy or prana from the bottom of the spine to the crown of the head.
- Feel the aliveness of body parts, hands, fingers, arms and legs; feel the energy radiate to every part of the body.
- Breathe in long and deep and breathe out even longer and deeper.
- Breathe in long and deep and hold the breath for a few seconds.
- Breathe out long and deep and hold the breath for a few seconds.

## *Abdominal Breathing*

In any comfortable posture, be aware of your breathing. Encourage yourself to make full use of the diaphragm by drawing air into the lowest and largest part of the lungs. As you inhale, be aware that the abdomen is rising. As you exhale, the abdomen is falling. The verbal instruction can follow: "Inhale: abdomen or belly out. Exhale: the abdomen or belly in." Make a note that during āsana practice, abdominal breathing is used throughout.

## *Full Yogic Breath*

In the full yogic breath, inhalation happens in three stages. First, the diaphragm moves downwards into the abdomen, drawing air into the lowest part of the lungs. Then, the intercostal muscles expand the rib cage and pull air into the middle part of the lungs. Lastly, air comes into the upper part of chest; this is called clavicular breathing. Sit in a cross-legged position. Inhale slowly, feel the abdomen expand first, then the rib cage, and finally, feel the air fill the upper chest. As you exhale, the air leaves the lower lung first, then the middle and lastly the top part.

# *Kapalabhati: "Shining Skull" Or "Fierce Breath"*

Kapalabhati is considered to be so cleansing to the entire system that, when practiced on a regular basis the practitioner's face shines with good health and radiance.

## *Method*

1. Sit in a cross-legged position, with your back straight and your head and spine erect. Take 2–3 deep abdominal breaths to prepare.
2. Contract the abdominal muscles, allowing the diaphragm to move up into the thoracic cavity and push the air out of the lung forcefully.
3. Passive inhalation takes place after deep and forceful contraction. The lungs automatically expand and inflate with air. Do not force the inhalation.
4. Continuously repeat the pumping quickly and follow with passive inhalation until a round is completed.
5. At the end of each round, allow 2–3 full yogic breaths, then hold breath for 30 seconds or up to 2 minutes.
6. Beginners start with 3 rounds with 20–30 pumps each and gradually increase to 5 rounds of 50–120 pumps.

# *Anuloma Viloma: Alternate Nostril Breathing*

This exercise helps calm the mind, making it lucid and steady, preparing for meditation. It purifies the nadis and practicing it helps store and control prana, vital energy. It balances the psychic system and makes the body light and the eyes shiny. It strengthens and cleanses the entire respiratory system. It helps balance the hemispheres of the brain. Because the breath naturally alternates between the 2 nostrils, changing approximately every 2 hours, practicing Anuloma Viloma helps balance "hot" sun-like right nostril and "cool" moon-like left nostril.

1. Sit cross-legged with your back straight and head and spine erect. Position your left hand in Chin Mudra (index finger touches middle finger) and your right hand in Vishnu Mudra (index and middle fingers fold into the palm while the thumb, ring finger and pinky extend). Breathe deeply for 2–3 breaths.
2. Inhale through both nostrils and bring the right hand to the nose and close the right nostril with the right thumb.
3. Exhale with the left nostril slowly and completely for 8 counts/seconds.
4. Inhale with the left nostril deeply for 4 counts/seconds.
5. Retain the breath with both nostrils closed with thumb and ring finger for 16 counts/seconds.
6. Exhale with the right nostril for 8 counts/seconds.
7. Inhale with the right nostril for 4 counts/seconds.
8. Retain the breath for 16 counts/seconds.

Repeat the process for at least three rounds, up to 10 rounds a day. As you become more advanced the "count" of the exercise may be increased, but always in a ratio of 1–4–2, for example, 4–16–8, 5–20–10, 6–24–12, 7–28–14, 8–32–16.

# Advanced Pranayama

Breathing exercises are practices that purify and strengthen the physical body as well as calm the mind. Steady practice of prānāyāma arouses the inner spiritual force and brings ecstatic joy, spiritual light and peace of mind. The body becomes strong and healthy, the voice becomes sweet and melodious, the nadis purify and the mind becomes one-pointed and prepared for dhāranā and dhyāna.

Here, we start to introduce bandhas as an integral part of and an essential part of advanced prānāyāma practice. They are practiced to awaken the potential psychic energy known as kundalini, which is said to reside in a coiled, dormant state at the base of the spine. The bandhas regulate the flow of prana (life force) within subtle energy channels known as nadis. Bandhas are a series of internal energy gates or centers within the subtle body which assists in the regulation of pranic flow.

The word bandha means lock. Bandhas are used along with mudras to lock and seal the prana into certain areas. When engaging in locks (holding the bandhas), energy is forced to flow through these pathways. We can then assimilate this energy on a cellular level as the prana bathes and feeds our subtle body and balances the gross nervous system. The three bandhas applied in advanced prānāyāma practice are discussed here. They are Moola Bandha, Uddiyana Bandha and Jalandhara Bandha.

Jalandhara Bandha and Uddiyana Bandha are engaged simultaneously during breath retention and this unites prana and apana. Engaging all three bandhas simultaneously is called Mahabandha.

1. **Moola Bandha** is the root lock and is located at the base of the spinal column. In males, the seat of the Moola Bandha is the perineal muscle which is located in front of the anus and behind the genitals. In females, it is located near the top of the cervix. A good way to understand the location is to hold the urge to urinate. When first practicing Moola Bandha consciously and gently contract the anus to engage the appropriate area. Only after you have practiced for a long time, will you be able to engage the necessary muscle.

2. **Uddiyana Bandha** is located 2 inches below the navel. To engage the Uddiyana Bandha, exhale fully and draw the intestines and the navel up towards the back so that the abdomen rests against the back of the body, high in the thoracic cavity.

3. **Jalandhara Bandha** is the chin lock. To engage it, extend the chin forward and then draw it back into the notch which is formed where the 2 clavicle bones meet: at the bony protrusions below the Adam's apple. Place the top of the tongue flat against the roof of the mouth and slide it back so that a vacuum is created in the back of the throat. At the same time press the chin firmly against the chest.

## *More Pranayama Techniques*

### *Surya Bedha*

1. With your right hand in Vishnu Mudra, close your left nostril.
2. Inhale through your right nostril.
3. Close both nostrils and retain your breath while applying Jalandhara Bandha, Moola Bandha and Uddiyana Bandha.
4. Hold your breath for as long as it is comfortable.
5. Release the head and release the bandhas.
6. Exhale through the left nostril. This is the end of one round. Repeat for up to 20 rounds.

### *Ujjayi*

Ujjayi is also called victorious breath. This unique form of breathing is performed by creating a soft sound in the back of throat while inhaling and exhaling through the nose. The swirling action is what creates the unique sound which has been described as wind in the trees, a distant ocean and a cobra.

1. Sit in the meditative position and close your mouth.
2. Inhale through both nostrils in a smooth uniform manner while partially closing the epiglottis in order to produce a soft sobbing sound of a sweet and uniform pitch.
3. At the end of the inhalation, close both your nostrils with your right hand in Vishnu Mudra and apply Moola Bandha and Jalandhara Bandha while holding your breath.
4. Exhale with the left nostril.
5. Then, inhale through the right nostril. This is end of one round. Repeat for up to 20 rounds.

### *Sheetkari*

Sheetkari purifies the blood, quenches thirst and cools the system.

1. Touch the tip of your tongue to the upper palate.
2. Inhale through your mouth.
3. Exhale through both of your nostrils.

### *Sheetali*

Sheetali purifies the blood, quenches thirst and cools the system.

1. Fold your tongue into a tube and protrude it between your lips.
2. Inhale through your mouth.
3. Exhale through both of your nostrils.

### *Bhastrika*

Kapalabhati and Bhastrika may appear similar, but Kapalabhati only uses the diaphragm while Bhastrika uses the entire respiratory system.

1.  Perform 10 and up to 30 rapid expulsions followed by a deep inhalation.

2.  Hold your breath and apply Moola Bandha and Jalandhara Bandha with your right hand in Vishnu Mudra.

3.  Exhale through your left nostril. This is the end of one round. Repeat for up to 10 rounds.

### Brahmari

1.  Inhale through the nose, producing a snoring sound.

2.  Exhale to produce a humming sound. Repeat for up to 10 rounds.

## BKS Iyengar 11-Step Practice Guide

Here, I would like to mention a systemic pranayama technique as taught by Guruji BKS Iyengar. This method is very practical and has been easily adopted by students for many years.

## Phase One—1/1 (Alternation of Nostrils with Rechaka/Puraka)

Prepare for prānāyāma

1.  Inhale through both your nostrils.

2.  Exhale through your left nostril long and deep (close your right nostril with your right thumb and let go of impurity via your left nostril; Guruji emphasized this all the time).

3.  Inhale through your left nostril.

4.  Exhale through your right nostril.

5.  Inhale through your right nostril.

6.  Repeat steps 2–5 twice.

7.  Exhale through your left nostril.

8.  This above process (1–7) completes 1 cycle and continues for a total of 12 cycles.

Take a few natural breaths after each cycle and make sure to use chips for counting (12 chips).

## Phase Two—1/1/1 (Alternation of Nostrils with Puraka/Rechaka/ Kumbhaka)

Prepare for prānāyāma

1.  Inhale through both your nostrils.

2.  Exhale through your left nostril long and deep (close your right nostril with your right thumb and let go of impurity via your left nostril; Guruji emphasized this all the time).

3.  Inhale through your left nostril.

4.  Retain the breath.

5.  Exhale through your right nostril.

6.  Inhale through your right nostril.

7.  Retain the breath.

8. Repeat steps 2–7 twice.

9. Exhale through your left nostril.

10. This above process (1–9) completes 1 cycle and continues for a total of 12 cycles.

Take a few natural breaths after each cycle and make sure to use chips for counting (12 chips).

## Phase Three—12/12/12 (Alternation of Nostrils with Puraka/Rechaka/Kumbhaka)

Prepare for prānāyāma

1. Inhale through both your nostrils.

2. Exhale through your left nostril long and deep (close your right nostril with your right thumb and let go of impurity via left nostril; Guruji emphasized this all the time).

3. Inhale through your left nostril for 12 counts.

4. Retain the breath for 12 counts.

5. Exhale through your right nostril for 12 counts.

6. Inhale through your right nostril for 12 counts.

7. Retain the breath for 12 counts.

8. Repeat steps 2–7 twice.

9. Exhale through your left nostril.

10. This above process (1–9) completes 1 cycle and continues for a total of 12 cycles.

Take a few natural breaths after each cycle and make sure to use chips for counting (12 chips).

## Phase Four—15/15/15 (Alternation of Nostrils with Puraka/Rechaka/Kumbhaka)

Prepare for prānāyāma

1. Inhale through both your nostrils.

2. Exhale through your left nostril long and deep (close your right nostril with your right thumb and let go of impurity via your left nostril; Guruji emphasized this all the time).

3. Inhale through your left nostril for 15 counts.

4. Retain your breath for 15 counts.

5. Exhale through your right nostril for 15 counts.

6. Inhale through your right nostril for 15 counts.

7. Retain the breath for 15 counts.

8. Repeat steps 2–7 twice.

9. Exhale through your left nostril.

10. This above process (1–9) completes 1 cycle and continues for a total of 12 cycles.

Take a few natural breaths after each cycle and make sure to use chips for counting (12 chips).

## *Phase Five—Sheetali and Sheetkari (Cooling) PrānāYāMa*

This prānāyāma inhalation is completed through the mouth only, without Jalandhara Bandha.

Prepare for prānāyāma with both hands on the knees

1. Inhale with curled tongue (U-shape) long and deep.
2. Exhale for 12 counts using Ujjayi breath.
3. Repeat steps 1–2 for 12 cycles.

Take a few natural breaths after each cycle and make sure to use chips for counting (12 chips).

## *Phase Six—Bhastrika and Kapalabhati (Fierce) PrānāYāMa*

Bhastrika means blow. Air is forcibly drawn in and out rhythmically. The sound is like that made by a blacksmith's bellows. Prepare for prānāyāma with both hands on the knees.

1. Inhale and exhale quickly and soundly for 4–30 blows.
2. Retain the breath briefly.
3. Exhale slowly. Take a few slow and deep Ujjayi breaths.
4. Repeat steps 1–4 for 12 cycles.

Take a few natural breaths after each cycle and make sure to use chips for counting (12 chips).

## *Phase Seven—18/18/18 (Alternation of Nostrils with Puraka/Rechaka/ Kumbhaka)*

Prepare for prānāyāma

1. Inhale through both your nostrils.
2. Exhale through your left nostril long and deep (close your right nostril with your right thumb and let go of impurity via your left nostril; Guruji emphasized this all the time).
3. Inhale through your left nostril for 18 counts.
4. Retain the breath for 18 counts.
5. Exhale through your right nostril for 18 counts.
6. Inhale through your right nostril for 18 counts.
7. Retain the breath for 18 counts.
8. Repeat steps 2–7 twice.
9. Finish by exhaling through your left nostril.
10. This above process (1-9) completes 1 cycle and continues for a total of 12 cycles.

Take a few natural breaths after each cycle and make sure to use chips for counting (12 chips).

## Phase Eight—18/18/24 (Alternation of Nostrils with Puraka/Rechaka/Kumbhaka)

Prepare for prānāyāma

1. Inhale through both your nostrils.
2. Exhale through your left nostril long and deep (close your right nostril with your right thumb and let go of impurity via your left nostril; Guruji emphasized this all the time).
3. Inhale through your left nostril for 18 counts.
4. Retain the breath for 24 counts.
5. Exhale through your right nostril for 18 counts.
6. Inhale through your right nostril for 18 counts.
7. Retain the breath for 24 counts.
8. Repeat steps 2–7 twice.
9. Exhale through your left nostril.
10. This above process (1–9) completes 1 cycle and continues for a total of 12 cycles.

Take a few natural breaths after each cycle and make sure to use chips for counting (12 chips).

## Phase Nine—18/18/30 (Alternation of Nostrils with Puraka/Rechaka/Kumbhaka)

Prepare for prānāyāma

1. Inhale through both your nostrils.
2. Exhale through your left nostril long and deep (close your right nostril with your right thumb and let go of impurity via your left nostril; Guruji emphasized this all the time).
3. Inhale through your left nostril for 18 counts.
4. Retain the breath for 30 counts.
5. Exhale through your right nostril for 18 counts.
6. Inhale through your right nostril for 18 counts.
7. Retain the breath for 30 counts.
8. Repeat steps 2–7 twice.
9. Exhale through your left nostril.
10. This above process (1–9) completes 1 cycle and continues for a total of 12 cycles.

Take a few natural breaths after each cycle and make sure to use chips for counting (12 chips).

## Phase Ten—24/24/24 (Alternation of Nostrils with Puraka/Rechaka/Kumbhaka)

Prepare for prānāyāma.

1. Inhale through both your nostrils.
2. Exhale through your left nostril long and deep (close your right nostril with your right thumb and let go of impurity via your left nostril; Guruji emphasized this all the time).
3. Inhale through your left nostril for 24 counts.
4. Retain the breath for 24 counts.
5. Exhale through your right nostril for 24 counts.
6. Inhale through your right nostril for 24 counts.
7. Retain the breath for 24 counts.
8. Repeat steps 2–7 twice.
9. Exhale through your left nostril.
10. This above process (1–9) completes 1 cycle and continues for a total of 12 cycles.

Take a few natural breaths after each cycle and make sure to use chips for counting (12 chips).

## Phase Eleven—24/24/30 (Alternation of Nostrils with Puraka/Rechaka/Kumbhaka)

Prepare for prānāyāma

1. Inhale through both your nostrils.
2. Exhale through your left nostril long and deep (close your right nostril with your right thumb and let go of impurity via your left nostril; Guruji emphasized this all the time).
3. Inhale through your left nostril for 24 counts.
4. Retain the breath for 30 counts.
5. Exhale through your right nostril for 24 counts.
6. through your right nostril for 24 counts.
7. Retain the breath for 30 counts.
8. Repeat steps 2–7 twice.
9. Exhale through your left nostril.
10. This above process (1–9) completes 1 cycle and continues for a total of 12 cycles.

Take a few natural breaths after each cycle and make sure to use chips for counting (12 chips).

# Kriya (Daily Cleansing)

The purpose of yogic cleansing exercises, known as kriyas, is to assist nature to remove waste products in the body. The *Hatha Yoga Pradipika*, which was written in ancient times, prescribes various kriyas. All kriyas are especially beneficial during fasting; they help to speed up the detoxification process. Fasting with kriyas is nature's cure for many diseases caused by toxins in the body.

## 1. Jala Neti: Water Nasal Cleansing

Neti is a technique for cleansing the nose, nasal passages and sinuses. It is important for maintaining freedom of breath and combating pollution. String, salt water and air are used to assist nature in cleansing the nasal passage and mucous membrane. They not only remove foreign matter but also prevent colds and keep the olfactory nerve healthy. Add a teaspoon of sea salt to a glass of lukewarm water and stir well. With the use of a neti pot, pour the salted water into one nostril until water comes out of the other nostril while keeping the head tilted sideways or backwards. If one nostril is blocked, raise the head and gently blow the excess water out of the nostrils. Repeat with the other nostril. Repeat this process 2–3 times with each nostril. It is important to remember not to inhale while pouring the water into the nostrils. Practice this method daily especially during allergy season. An alternative method is to raise the head to allow the salted water to flow down into the throat and out of mouth. Do not try to inhale while pouring it; this brings an unpleasant sensation. Just allow the water to flow to the mouth naturally by keeping the head tilted back, and then spit the water out.

## 2. Nauli: Abdominal Churning

To practice Nauli, turn the intestines of the abdomen to the right and left or up and down like the slow motion of a small eddy in the river. It is considered the crown of hatha yoga practices; it drives away the dullness of the gastric fire, increases the digestive power, produces a pleasing sensation and diminishes the diseases associated with digestion. Combined with Uddiyana Bandha, Nauli is the best exercise for strengthening the abdominal muscles and assisting in the elimination of waste products and removing sluggishness of the stomach, intestines and livers. In Nauli practice, the manipulation of these muscles, increases circulation.

**Uddiyana Bandha practice:** In a standing position, place your hands firmly on your thighs, with your legs apart and your body bent lightly forward. Forcefully exhale. Draw the navel and intestines inwards and upwards, so that the abdomen rests against the back of the body high in the thoracic cavity. Hold the abdomen in the raised position as long as possible without inhaling. This can be repeated 5–8 times with brief intervals to rest. This can be practiced daily.

**Nauli practice:** While holding Uddiyana Bandha, contract the left and right sides of the abdomen. This brings the abdominal muscles into a vertical line. After you have mastered the central Nauli, the next step is to practice the up-to-down and the side-to-side churning abdomen.

Caution: This should not be practiced by pregnant women or by a person who has abdominal cramps.

## 3. Agni Sara: Fire Purification

While holding Uddiyana Bandha and without inhaling, relax the abdominal muscles and draw them inward in quick succession. For one round do 5–10 pumps in this manner. Practice 3–5 rounds daily.

## 4. Kapalabhati: Cleansing of Lungs and Bronchial Tubes

Kapalabhati is usually practiced along with prānāyāma. It is an exercise for the purification of the nasal passages, bronchial tubes and lungs. It is the best exercise to stimulate every tissue in the body. During and after practice, you may experience a particular joy, especially in the spinal centers. When the vital nerve system is stimulated through this exercise, the entire spine will be like a live wire and one can experience the movement of nerve current. Great quantities of carbon dioxide gas are eliminated, while intake of oxygen makes the blood richer and renews the body tissues. The constant movement of the diaphragm acts as a stimulant to the stomach, liver, intestines and pancreas.

Kapalabhati — "shining skull" or "fierce breath" — is considered to be so cleansing to the entire system that when practiced on a regular basis the practitioner's face shines with good health and radiance.

1. Sit in a cross-legged position, with your back straight and your head and spine erect. Take 2–3 deep abdominal breaths to prepare.

2. Contract the abdominal muscles, allowing the diaphragm to move up into the thoracic cavity and forcefully push the air out of your lungs.

3. After the deep and forceful contraction, passive inhalation will take place. The lungs will automatically expand and inflate with air. Do not force the inhalation.

# Chapter 5

# ASANA PRACTICE AND THE IMPORTANCE OF MAINTAINING DIGESTIVE HEALTH

## Introduction and the Digestive Process

Many of the digestive organs, namely the esophagus, stomach, small intestine and large intestine, are hollow, to permit the free passage of food mixed with digestive juices. The accessory organs, the liver, kidneys, spleen and pancreas, are solid. This mixture of textures creates a diverse reaction when they press against each other during yogasanas.

### The Digestive System

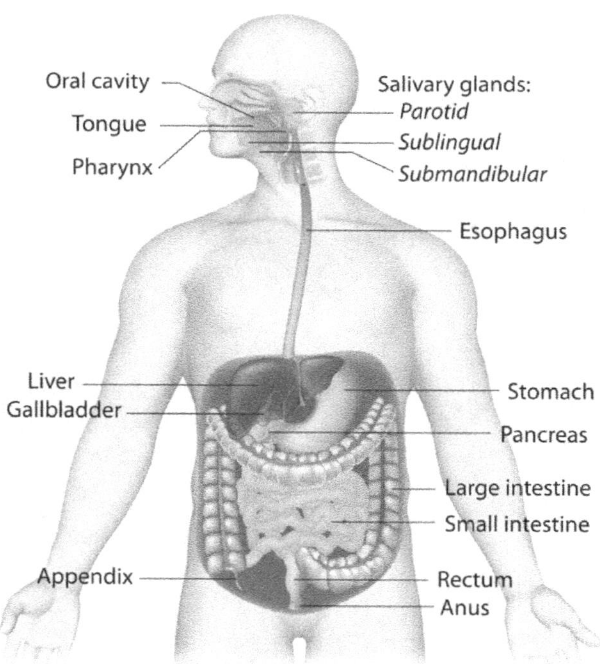

The inverted poses, twists and forward-bending poses reposition the digestive organs. Holding these poses longer and deepening your breath is most beneficial to digestion. It is wonderful to know yourself so well that you are able to breathe into each individual organ. This repositioning commonly creates peristaltic motion and accompanying sounds during these poses. This is especially true during Supported Shoulder Stand. (Often the class sounds like a frog serenade following a rainstorm!) Encourage these sounds when practicing on your own. Whatever motion brought it up, repeat it, going into and out of the motion several times until the internal serenade is complete.

Constipation and irregular bowel movements are aggravated by irregular lifestyles. The most effective therapy to address this immediately is to regulate eating and sleeping habits. Regular practice of yogasana will help you begin to understand your own body's language. The body develops its own sensitivity and knows whether the food you eat is "right" or not. Your internal clock regulates your schedule precisely, and your body lets you know if you're exercising too much, sleeping too much and so forth.

The next step is to heighten your sensitivity to increase your self-observation skills. This will help you detect foods that are indigestible to your system. These may include leftovers held over 24 hours that lose their lifeforce, overcooked foods, processed foods and sugar.

The third step is to develop humility and reverence for the process of growing, gathering, harvesting and preparing food. Cultivate thankfulness for each person and the forces of nature that created the blessing of the food that will soon become your body. By blessing your food, you will find yourself drawn to eating foods that want to become your body.

## Ayurveda Medicine and Recommendations

### Introduction to Ayurveda Medicine

Ayurveda, which literally means "the science of life," is the natural healing system used throughout India. Ayurveda was originally known to have been first developed and established by the great sages who developed India's original systems of meditation and yoga.

The study of Ayurveda includes herbal medicine, dietetics, body work, surgery, psychology and spirituality. It deals not only with medical science but also with the social, ethical, intellectual and spiritual life of man. Ayurveda amalgamates the accuracy of science and the sublimity of philosophy, poetry and art.

According to Ayurveda, the human body is composed of five fundamental elements called Panchamahabhootas (earth, water, fire, air and ether) three doshas, seven dhatus (tissues) and three malas. The doshas govern the physio-chemical and physiological activities of the body, while the dhatus enter into the formation of a basic structure of a body cell, thereby performing some specific actions. The malas are impurities partly excreted in a modified form after serving their physiological functions. These three elements are said to be in a dynamic equilibrium with each other for the maintenance of health. Any imbalance of their relative importance in the body results in disease and illness.

Today, an estimated 300,000 ayurvedic physicians practice in India, often in close conjunction with doctors trained in Western, conventional medicine or in homeopathy. Ayurvedic practitioners teach patients to understand their unique bodily constitutions and show them how to use diet, massage, herbs and lifestyle adjustments to harmonize body, mind and spirit. In recent years, a more science-savvy take on Ayurveda has spread to distant parts of the world, where it has begun to flourish alongside other holistic, patient-oriented, natural, non-invasive medical systems such as traditional Chinese medicine.

According to Ayurveda, every living creature is composed of soul, mind and body. It is the compound of these three elements that constitutes the science of life. Ayurveda is a holistic system of medicine from India that uses a constitutional model. Its aim is to provide guidance regarding food and lifestyle so that healthy people can stay healthy and folks with health challenges can improve their health.

## Unique Aspects of Ayurveda

1. Its recommendations will often be different for each person regarding which foods and which lifestyle they should follow to be completely healthy. This is due to its use of a constitutional model.
2. Everything in Ayurveda is validated by observation, inquiry, direct examination and knowledge derived from the ancient texts. It understands that there are energetic forces that influence nature and human beings.
3. These forces are called the Tridoshas.
4. Because Ayurveda sees a strong connection between the mind and the body, a huge amount of information is available regarding this relationship.

## Origin

Ayurveda is an intricate system of healing that originated in India thousands of years ago. We find historical evidence of Ayurveda in the ancient books of wisdom known as the vedas. The *Rig Veda* mentions over 60 preparations that can be used to assist an individual in overcoming various ailments. The *Rig Veda* was written over 6,000 years ago, but really Ayurveda has been around even longer than that. What we see is that Ayurveda is more than just a medical system. It is a Science of Life. We are all part and parcel of nature. Just as animals and plants live in harmony with nature and utilize the Laws of Nature to create health and balance within their beings, we, too, adhere to these very same principles. Therefore, it is fair to say that Ayurveda is a system that helps maintain health in a person by using the inherent principles of nature to bring the individual back into equilibrium with their true self. In essence, Ayurveda has been in existence since the beginning of time because we have always been governed by nature's laws.

## Meaning

Ayurveda is made up of two Sanskrit words: Ayu which means life and Veda which means knowledge of. To know about life is Ayurveda. However, to fully comprehend the vast scope of Ayurveda, let us first define "Ayu" or life. According to the ancient Ayurvedic scholar Charaka, "ayu" comprises four essential parts: mind, body, senses and the soul.

## Mind, Body and Senses

We tend to identify most with our physical bodies; yet, there is more to us then what meets the eye. Underlying our physical structure is the mind, which not only controls our thought processes but helps assist us in carrying out day-to-day activities such as respiration, circulation, digestion and elimination. The mind and the body work in conjunction with one another to regulate our physiology. For the mind to act appropriately to assist the physical body, we must use our senses as information gatherers. We can think of the mind as a computer and the senses as the data which gets entered into the computer. Smell and taste are two important senses that aid in the digestive process. When the mind registers that a particular food is entering the gastrointestinal tract, it directs the body to act accordingly by releasing various digestive enzymes. However, if we overindulge our taste buds with too much of a certain taste, such as sweet, we may find that the ability of the mind to perceive the sweet taste is impaired and the body is thus challenged in its ability to process sweet food. Maintaining the clarity of our senses is an essential part of allowing the mind and body to integrate their functions and help in keeping us healthy and happy individuals.

## Soul

Ayurveda also sees that before we exist in the physical form with the help of the mind and senses, we exist in a subtler form known as the soul. The ancient seers of India believed that we were composed of a certain energetic essence that precluded the inhabitance of our physical entity. In fact, they hypothesized that we may indeed occupy many physical bodies throughout the course of time but that our underlying self or soul remains unchanged. What we see to help illustrate this concept is what transpires at the time of death. When the time nears for an individual to leave the physical body, many of his/her desires will cease to be present. As the soul no longer identifies with the body, the desire to eat food or indulge in a particular activity that used to be a great source of satisfaction for that person drops by the wayside. In fact, many individuals have been documented to experience the sensation of being "out of their bodies." These are just a few examples of how we are made up of these four components that we call life.

## Principles

Now that we have a better understanding of what comprises life, let's look at some of the principles of Ayurveda and how they might affect us. In Ayurveda, we view a person as a unique individual made up of five primary elements. The elements are ether (space), air, fire, water and earth. Just as in nature, we too have these five elements in us. When any of these elements are present in the environment, they will, in turn, have an influence on us. The foods we eat and the weather are just two examples of the presence of these elements.

While we are a composite of these five primary elements, certain elements are seen to have an ability to combine to create various physiological functions. Ether and air combine to form what is known in

Ayurveda as the Vata dosha. Vata governs the principle of movement and can, therefore, be considered the force that directs nerve impulses, circulation, respiration and elimination. Fire and water are the elements that combine to form the Pitta dosha. The Pitta dosha is the process of transformation or metabolism. The transformation of foods into nutrients that our bodies can assimilate is an example of a Pitta function. Pitta is responsible for metabolism in the organ and tissue systems and cellular metabolism. Finally, it is predominantly the water and earth elements which combine to form the Kapha dosha. Kapha is what is responsible for growth, adding structure unit by unit. Another function of the Kapha dosha is to offer protection. Cerebral-spinal fluid protects the brain and spinal column and is a type of Kapha found in the body. Also, the mucosal lining of the stomach is another example of the Kapha dosha protecting the tissues. We are all made up of unique proportions of Vata, Pitta and Kapha. The ratios of the doshas vary in each individual, because of which Ayurveda sees each person as a special mixture that accounts for our diversity.

Ayurveda gives us a model to look at each individual as a unique makeup of the three doshas and to thereby design treatment protocols that specifically address a person's health challenges. When any of the doshas (Vata, Pitta or Kapha) accumulate, Ayurveda will suggest specific lifestyle and nutritional guidelines to assist the individual in reducing the dosha that has become excessive. Certain herbal supplements may also be suggested to hasten the healing process. If toxins abound in the body, then a cleansing process known as Pancha Karma (five therapeutic cleansing procedures) is recommended to eliminate them.

## Conclusion

This understanding that we are all unique individuals enables Ayurveda to address not only specific health concerns but also explains why one person responds differently than another. We hope that you will continue to explore Ayurveda to enhance your health and to gain further insights into this miracle we call life.

## Five Elements of the Cosmos

- **Earth:** heaviness, matter, denseness, coldness, groundedness of mind, skeletal structure of body
- **Water:** heaviness, coldness, moistness, fluidity in body, nourishment, emotion/love/compassion
- **Fire:** heat, transformation, warmth, metabolization, power of perception
- **Air:** motion, mobility, coldness, lightness, dryness, movement, thoughts in mind
- **Ether:** space, light, flow, mobile, connect

## The Three Doshas—Prakriti and Vikriti

- **Vata (air and ether):** dry, cold, light, thin and long figure, long arms; when off-balance—not grounded, not responsible, emotional, panic, fear, constipation
- **Pitta (fire and water):** hot, light, moist, medium and defined figure, leader, sharp; when off-balance—rashes, intense, angry, jealousy, acidic, sores
- **Kapha (earth and water):** heavy, cold, moist, bigger structure, rounder face, large eyes, thick hair; when off-balance—lethargic, inertial, weight gain, not motivated

## Function of Digestion

- **Agni or enzymes:** assist the digestion and assimilation of food, located in digestive track, liver and seven tissues.
- **Ama:** a form of liquid sludge, lodges in parts of the body blocking the channels, a product of improperly digested food and drink.

## Three Mental States—"Gunas"

- **Sattva:** balance, serenity, joy, health, productivity, happiness, sharpness
- **Rajas:** energy, activity, motion, excitement
- **Tamas:** inertia, lethargy, laziness, heaviness

## Six Tastes of Food/Herb

1. Sweet—earth/water (cold): grains, fruit, sugar, starch
2. Salty—water/fire (hot): seaweed, table salt
3. Sour—earth/fire (hot): fermented food and acidic fruit
4. Pungent—fire/air (hot): hot spices, cayenne, ginger
5. Bitter—air/ether (cold): goldenseal, gentian
6. Astringent—earth/air (cold): herbs containing tannins like alum or witch hazel

## Recommendations

- Always respect your food and begin each meal by giving thanks for it. Or simply take 3–5 breaths with your eyes closed. This prepares the body to receive food.
- Maintain a peaceful attitude during meals and avoid watching TV, reading and indulging in heated discussions.
- The attitude with which one eats food is just as important as the food being eaten. Being obsessive about food is just as disruptive as disregarding it. Take a moment before eating to relax and become aware that you are going to give your system food. Saying grace is a way to set this state of mind.
- The main meal should be eaten between 10 am and 2 pm, while the digestive fire is the highest and strongest.
- Do not eat after sunset.
- Eat at a moderate pace (not too fast or too slow), until you are three-fourths full. After eating, you should not feel heavy. Overeating causes lots of problems, even diseases.
- Do not drink excessive amounts of fluid during the meal; it dilutes the digestive enzymes.
- Avoid drinking ice-cold water; it dampens agni, the digestive fire. A half cup at room temperature or hot water is average. Allow three hours between meals to digest.
- Eat food that is prepared with good and positive energy. The energy of the cook is always in the food.

- Salads and greens are best consumed after other foods as the bitterness cuts the digestive fluids.
- Eat fruit alone or before other food, otherwise it sits and ferments. Cooking fruits makes them easier to digest for those who have a weak digestive system. Make sure to eat melon alone, not even with other fruits.
- Do not consume milk with fruit. Have it alone or with starchy foods.
- Do not combine concentrated proteins, for example beans, nuts, fish, or dairy.
- Eat only fresh food; avoid pre-made, canned, frozen or leftover food. Fresh foods have the highest prana.
- Have all six tastes in each meal. This helps to achieve balance and prevent unusual cravings.
- Let the eaten food digest before starting another activity—read or take a slow walk for a few minutes. Or if you do not have time, then take 3–5 slow breaths to acknowledge the completion of eating.
- Observe silence when eating alone.
- Do not eat when you are angry.
- Do not eat food that is too hot or too cold.
- Do not force yourself to eat something you do not like and do not eat only those foods you like the most. Eat at least one raw dish in each meal to maintain the blood alkaline level.
- Clean your mouth before eating.
- Eat slowly and savor your food.
- Eat moderately and at fixed times. Eat as little processed food as possible.
- Foods are best consumed when cooked lightly.
- Try not to eat large meals late at night.
- Eat to live, do not live to eat.
- Take lemon and honey in the morning to purify the blood.
- Do not practice āsana immediately after a meal or when you are hungry.
- Try to sit in Vijra Āsana (sit on your heels with your knees and feet together) for 10 minutes after a meal.
- Do not become a slave to food and drink.
- Try to fast once a week.
- Remember God dwells in all foods.

# Ayurveda Yoga

Understanding imbalances and balances for each dosha can help create focus during yoga practice that is healing for each individual constitution.

## Ayurveda Yoga Basics for the Vatha Dosha

Emotions and abilities—fear, insecurity, anxiety, creativity, flexibility

Imbalance—insomnia, worries, gas, constipation, underweight, cracking joints

Main sites—colon, pelvic cavity, bones, brain, skin

- It is important to warm up the joints sufficiently before practice. Pranayama—Ujiayi, full yogic breath, abdominal breath, nadi shodhana, so-hum staying in the gap between two breaths. Focus more on retention of breath gradually and do not force.
- Strengthening—poses that build strength, stability and flexibility. Grounding—always brings awareness to grounding through feet, stability in each pose, focusing on lower chakra poses.
- Open and strengthen the pelvic floor, focus on poses that increase the prana to the hips. Take the femurs back and ground them in the hip socket.
- Strengthen the back of the neck, practice poses that release and strengthen the back of the neck muscles.
- Gentleness—be mindful not to strain.
- Sufficient rest is needed between poses. Hatha yoga is more appropriate. Practice the anti-rheumatic group of poses designed to warm up every joint in the body and release excess Vatha.

## Ayurveda Yoga Basics for the Pitta Dosha

Emotion and abilities—ambition, irritability, jealousy, anger, aggressiveness, frustration, concentration, a thirst for knowledge, determination, strength

Imbalance—Diarrhea, ulcers, acid indigestion, migraine headache, inflammatory problems, skin rashes, red eyes

Main sites—liver, spleen, heart, brain, blood, eyes, skin, small intestine, secretion, sweat

Warm-up the abdominal area before practice when Pitta is elevated. When breathing, focus on longer exhalation then inhalation, slow gentle breath around the solar plexus, Sitali and Sitakari (cooling breaths), Chandra Bhedana (left nostril breath), Anuloma pranayama and Bahir Kumbhaka in Ujjayi (external retention).

- Balance effort with surrender through non-competitive practice without trying to achieve the perfect pose.
- Balance inaction with action. Rest between poses. Softness—soften temples, eyes and mind. Bring love, calmness and acceptance to practice.
- Open the navel area, focus on poses that open the navel and release revitalizing energy around the liver.
- Twists detoxify the liver, alleviate anger and relieve exhaustion.
- Coolness—practice in a well-ventilated room, complete the session with forward bends and twists.
- Practice the digestive and abdominal group poses designed to strengthen the digestive system and eliminate energy that is blocked in the abdominal area. Other adjustments for Pitta include taking gaze downward, inward, lifting the skull, lengthening the neck and letting the entire rib cage area soften.

- Perform only to 60 percent of your ability in each pose.

# Ayurveda Yoga Basics for the Kapha Dosha

Emotions and abilities—attachment, greed, love, calmness, faith, lethargy

Imbalances—sinus and bronchial congestion, slow digestion, excess weight, sluggishness, asthma, diabetes, cold, cough, dullness of mind, greed, depression

Main sites—lymph nodes, breast tissues, chest, lungs, sinus, mouth, throat

- Do vigorous energizing warm-up if Kapha is elevated. Increase heart rate—choose challenging asanas and short rests.
- Do rapid sun salutation.
- Breathing—bring breath all the way to upper chest, Ujjayi pranayama, Kapalabhati, Surya Bhedana (right nostril breath), Bhastrika and Bhramari (humming breath).
- Open chest pose that invites the arms held overhead.
- Lift the energy of the pelvic floor up to the chest and head.
- Lift inner ankles in standing poses, engage upper thighs to lift and inner ankles to bring energy to each pose.
- Backbends and twists help move energy into stomach and chest.
- Do vigorous standing poses, energizing in each pose.
- Practice energy postures so one can obtain stagnant energy to move upward and release energy block in the spine, which activates the lungs.

# Yoga Diet

## *Introduction*

We are what we eat, claims the popular adage. Add to this, the knowledge that what you need to eat is not elaborate menus with unavailable and exotic ingredients, but simple home cooked food using regional and seasonally available ingredients that suit your constitution. Food is necessary for our physical well-being and it also affects the subtle aspects of our mind and our energy. A natural yogic diet is pure and "sattvic" and is based on fresh, light, nutritious food such as fruits, grains and vegetables. It keeps the body lean and limber and the mind clear and sharp, making it most suitable for yoga practice. It also provides the subtle energy, the prana, with the best possible guarantee of physical and mental health and brings harmony and vitality to the body and the mind.

A yogic diet is simple and the most natural. The sun, air, soil and water combine to produce the fruits of the earth, namely fruits, vegetables, legumes, nuts and seeds. Based on our anatomical and physiological nature, these products should be the main sources of our bodily needs. Our body, teeth and intestines are very different from those of carnivores.

Ahimsa "non-violence" is among the highest laws in yogic philosophy and cannot be disregarded when we grow spiritually. For the yogi, all life is sacred and every creature is a living entity. Once you become conscious of where your food comes from and how it affects you, your mind will gradually open and you will realize that all creatures are as divine as you are.

## The Three Gunas (Qualities of Food)

In the un-manifested universe, energy has three qualities, known as gunas, that exist together in equilibrium:

- Sattva (purity)
- Rājas (activity, passion and the process of change)
- Tamas (darkness and inertia)

The three gunas encompass all existence and all actions. Even among people, one of the three gunas plays a dominant role and is reflected in all that we do and think. Only in the enlightened state are gunas completely transcended. In yoga philosophy, the mind is formed from the subtle aspects or essence of food. If the food is pure, it brings inner peace to the body and mind and encourages spiritual progress. All of nature, including diet, is categorized into three qualities or gunas: sattva, rājas, and tamas. Yogis believe that not only are you what you eat but also the foods you eat reflect your own level of mental and spiritual purity. Yogic diet is based on sattvic foods.

## Sattvic Food

Pure foods that increase vitality, energy, health and joy and are delicious, wholesome, substantial and agreeable are sattvic. Such foods supply maximum energy and increase strength and endurance. Sattvic foods are fresh, as natural as possible, organically grown and do not use preservatives and artificial flavors. A sattvic diet is the purest and most suitable one for any serious yoga student and spiritual aspirant. It nourishes the body and maintains it in a peaceful state. It calms and purifies the mind, enabling one to function at one's maximum potential. A sattvic diet leads to a peaceful mind and a healthy body with a balanced flow of energy between them. Sattvic foods include grains, whole wheat bread, fresh fruits and vegetables, legumes, nuts, seeds, sprouted seeds and herb teas. Some sattvic grains are corn, barley, wheat, unpolished rice, oats, millet and quinoa. Some sattvic protein foods are nuts and seeds. Sattvic fruits are fresh, dried or pure fresh juice. Sattvic herbs are used for seasoning and teas. Some natural sweeteners are honey, molasses, maple syrup and apple juice concentrate; they are much better than processed sugar or sugar substitutes. Dairy products are part of the traditional yogic diet. However, many modern dairy practices abuse animals or feed them food laced with hormones and antibiotics. Dairy products also intensify the production of mucus and interfere with the natural flow of breath. So, include them in your diet only if you are sure the source is reliable.

## Rājasic Food

Rājasic foods are excessively hot, pungent, bitter, sour, dry and salty. They destroy the mind-body equilibrium, feeding the body at the expense of the mind. Too much rājasic food overstimulates the body and makes the mind restless and uncontrollable. Rājasic foods increase lust, anger, greed, selfishness, violence and egoism. They include coffee, tea, tobacco, all stimulants, refined sugar, soft drinks, spices and highly seasoned food.

## Tamasic Food

Tamasic food makes a person dull, inert and lazy. It fills the mind with darkness and decreases creativity and spirituality. Abandoning tamasic food is the first positive lifestyle change you can make. Eating excessive amounts of sattvic food (overeating) becomes tamasic. Tamasic foods include meats, fish and all intoxicants (alcohols, illegal drugs). They also include stale, decomposed, unclean and overripe fruits, food that is fermented, burned, fried, barbecued and reheated many times. It also includes foods containing preservatives (canned and processed foods).

# Ayurveda Dietary Guidelines for Efficient Yoga Practice

Yoga and Ayurveda are ancient sciences rooted in India, between 4,000 and 5,000 years old. They are related and support each other. Ayurveda means the knowledge of daily living or life; it is a holistic system which recognizes that humans are made of the same elements and forces of nature as the rest of creation: earth, fire, water, air and ether (space). Although it has a philosophical and spiritual basis, it focuses on physical health. Yoga is a spiritual system for the individual to transcend the material world and realize the true Self and to obtain super consciousness. Yoga includes practices for physical health, because without them it becomes difficult to focus on spiritual matters.

Ayurvedic doctors often prescribe yoga practice for healing while yogis use Ayurveda to help balance their mind and body, as support for their yoga practice. Many of the approaches taken by yoga and Ayurveda towards nutrition are, therefore, in agreement. However, there are some differences. For example, as the aim of yoga is to transcend the body through the increase in prana (life force), a yogic diet traditionally emphasizes more raw foods, while an ayurvedic diet emphasizes more cooked foods, particularly for certain constitution types or doshas. Also, a yogic diet focuses on sattvic food: food that brings peace to the mind and purifies the body. These are fresh foods with naturally sweet tastes, such as fruits, vegetables, grains and ghee (clarified butter). Rājasic foods, such as onion, garlic, hot spices, coffee and black tea, are over-stimulating and are avoided. However, according to Ayurveda, some of these foods in moderation are sometimes acceptable or recommended for certain constitution types. Tamasic food, which dulls the mind and leads to stagnation in the body are also avoided by yogis. Fried, overly processed, stale and heavy foods like meat, cheese, or heavy sweets fall into this category. Again, according to Ayurveda, some of these can be tolerated in small amounts by certain constitutions.

According to Ayurveda, the proper functioning of the digestive system is the most important factor in health. Ayurveda sees most illnesses as the result of impaired digestion, which can include absorption and elimination. When the digestive system is out of balance and foods are not properly digested, the result is gas, bloating, irritation, difficulty waking in the morning and constipation. Nutrients are not absorbed and undigested food accumulates in the colon, becoming a breeding ground for yeast infections and toxins. Undigested foods turn into a toxic substance called ama. The ama is the root cause of most problems in the body. Properly digested foods create nutritional essence. The health of the immune system determines whether diseases are warded off.

Ayurveda notes that there is a sap-like substance in the body called ojas that coats the immune system and protects it from diseases. If the agni (the fire in the body) is too low or too high, the life sap will be diminished. Just like a tree that produces sap over a bruise in its bark to protect and heal the bruise, our life sap (ojas) protects and heals us from illness. Overeating is one of the most common causes of suppressed agni, the digestive fire. Excessive agni can also cause problems, although this is not as common; it results from eating overly hot food, repressed anger and going for prolonged periods without eating. Too much dryness or too much heat and fire eat away the life sap. A weak immune system is the cause of all illnesses, from colds to multiple sclerosis to AIDS. To heal and maintain a good immune system, one needs adequate rest and pure sattvic foods and herbs that specifically rebuild the ojas. By eating small and simple meals, we can rebalance the agni. Supplements to the diet such as ginger tea, lemon or lime in water, or a spice mixture of ground cumin, coriander and fennel can help.

Ayurveda uses taste as an energetic classification for food as well as the heating/cooling action and post-digestive effects. These classifications are the result of the accumulation of knowledge over several thousand years. Different tastes arise owing to different combinations of the five elements, just like the different doshas (constitutional types). The tastes are simple ways to classify chemical and enzyme responses in the body to different substances. They have different effects on metabolism and will affect different people differently. The six tastes are sweet, salty, sour, bitter, astringent and pungent.

- Vata type: sweet, sour and salty
- Pitta type: sweet, bitter and astringent
- Kapha type: pungent, bitter and astringent

## *Fundamentals of Nutrition*
## *Eating for Wellness: The Yogic Diet*

Consider:

- What role does the food you eat play in your overall wellness?
- Why do you choose to eat what you do?
- What influences your eating habits?
- How is diet related to the Yogic Lifestyle?

### *Understand How Food Is Associated with Every Dimension of Wellness*

- Physical: physiological nourishment
- Emotional: affects feelings
- Social: used for celebrations
- Intellectual: forming decisions regarding selections
- Spiritual: used with rituals
- Environmental: food quantity and quality concepts
- Occupational: economic relationships, obtaining and using food

## *Studies Reveal 6 Shortfalls in Our Eating Habits*

1. Too few fruits and vegetables
2. Too little fiber
3. Too much fat (animal/saturated)
4. Too many refined sugars
5. Too much food overall
6. Inadequate water intake

## *Changing Our Diets*

The goal of promoting wellness can be accomplished by consuming

- Large amounts of fresh fruits/veggies
- Whole grain products
- Minimally processed foods
- Low saturated fat/animal protein
- Low refined sugars
- Lots of water
- Organic and local food

# Yogic Diet and Nutritional Basics

- Besides being responsible for building our physical body, the foods we eat profoundly affect our mind. For maximum body–mind efficiency and complete spiritual awareness, yoga advocates a lactovegetarian diet. This is an integral part of the yogic lifestyle.
- The yogi is concerned with the subtle effect that food has on his mind and astral body.
- The yogi prefers foods that calm the mind and sharpen the intellect.
- Someone serious about yoga would avoid meats, fish, eggs, onions, garlic, coffee, tea (except herbal), alcohol and drugs.

## *Nutrition Basics*

Principles of a healthy diet:

- Balance among carbs/fat/protein
- Variety of foods from different sources
- Moderation achieved through a mix of macronutrients (protein, carbohydrates, fats, water) and micronutrients (vitamins and minerals)

## *Nutrition Basics*

1. Carbohydrates (50–65 percent of total calories): provide energy, fiber, sweetener. Choose whole grain, unrefined, natural sources.

2. Protein (0.8 g/kg healthy body weight): many functions, including tissue formation and repair, fluid balance, immunity, hormone and enzymes.

   Plant protein: fiber, vitamins, minerals, unsaturated fatty acids Animal: cholesterol, saturated fatty acids, too much protein Complementary protein: beans (legumes), grains, nuts/seeds, vegetables

3. Fats (< 30 percent of total calories): provide energy, insulation, protection

   Essential fatty acids: immune function, hormone production, cell membranes, vision, cardiovascular health

   Saturated versus unsaturated fatty acids: choose unsaturated, avoid hydrogenated oils, animal fat, coconut and palm oils

   Good fats: nuts, seeds, avocado, olive

4. Vitamins and minerals

**Vitamins:**

- composed of carbon and other elements
- must be obtained from diet
- are essential to at least one vital process
- are found in nearly all foods, particularly fruits and vegetables

**Minerals:**

- composed of elements other than carbon
- serve important structural, electrical and chemical roles in the body

# Chapter 6

# YOGA CHIKITSA—AN INTRODUCTION TO YOGA THERAPY

Yoga therapy is based on the ancient principles of chikitsa krama (therapeutic orientation), which is derived from the yoga tradition of Patanjali and the Ayurvedic system of health, both of which, in turn, derive from the Sankhya and Upanishadic traditions of Vedic India.

Yoga chikitsa is a remedial tradition, based on the recognition that our physical condition, emotional states, attitudes, dietary and behavioral patterns, lifestyle and personal associations and the environment in which we live and work are intimately linked to each other and to our health.

According to yoga theory, we live within a framework of constant change (parinama) and within this framework, develop conditioned patterns (samskaras) that are present in every dimension of our lives and that influence our perceptions, thoughts, attitudes and behavior at every level. The good news is that because nothing is static, our condition will inevitably change. The salient question is, will it change for the better or for worse? Our challenge is to influence the direction of change for the better. This challenge is complicated by those patterns, often operating beneath the level of our conscious awareness, that influence our action. We may heal the body through some medical or alternate healing modality, but unless there is transformation at the level of our deep patterns, we may end up re-creating the same or similar conditions again.

Yoga chikitsa is the art of tapping the resources deep within us to heal ourselves. The belief that healing is a natural process goes along with a recognition that our attitudes and behavior can create conditions in our system—structurally, physiologically and psychologically—that inhibit that natural process. The allopathic physician's orientation is to treat the person. In yoga therapy, we are first and foremost seeking to change attitudes and actions that inhibit the natural healing process. The ideal is to develop the mind so that it can lead us on a path to improve the quality of life. According to ancient teachings, the main goal of yoga is to influence the state of mind. Our goal is first of all to help people feel better about themselves, gain more clarity about their lives, help them prioritize and become more effective in their actions and, perhaps most important, connect to a deeper source with themselves. I was taught: "To the extent that we inference the mind, we influence the entire system and to that extent, the person is better."

### *Dukha Samyoga Viyoga Yogaha*
### *"Yoga is separating from identification with suffering"*

There are two essential elements in this process: Viyoga and Samyoga. Viyoga literally means "separation." In the context of yoga therapy, Viyoga refers to the process of separating ourselves from whatever is undesirable in our lives. As an eliminative process, it involves the purification of both mind and body. It also involves letting go of unhealthy attachments, giving up self-destructive behavior and breaking detrimental relationships.

Samyoga literally means "linking together." In the context of yoga therapy, Samyoga refers to the process of linking to the positive and productive in our lives. It involves the development of mental qualities such as kindness, courage, patience and compassion. It also involves establishing appropriate priorities, practicing virtues and cultivating positive relationships.

The work of yoga therapy can be called "kayakalpa." This expression, from Ayurveda, is often presented as a science of immortality. In fact, kayakalpa refers literally to the reorganization, reconstruction and rejuvenation of our mind and body through practice. It involves a progressive reintegration of the entire system and a creation of harmony in every aspect of our lives.

Yoga therapy uses yoga postures, breathing exercises, meditation and guided imagery to improve mental and physical health. The holistic focus of yoga therapy encourages the integration of mind, body and spirit. Modern yoga therapy covers a broad range of therapeutic modalities, incorporating elements from both physical therapy and psychotherapy.

Yoga therapy may be defined as the application of yogic principles to a person with the objective of achieving a spiritual, psychological or physiological goal. Yoga therapy respects individual differences in age, culture, religion, philosophy, occupation and mental and physical health.

Yoga comprises a wide range of mind/body practices, from postural and breathing exercises to deep relaxation and meditation. Yoga therapy tailors these to the health needs of the individual. It helps to promote all-round positive health, as well as assisting particular medical conditions.

The yogic breath, which involves controlled and mindful breathing, increases lung capacity making it effective in managing chronic respiratory problems, like asthma. It also "detoxifies the body by flooding it with healing oxygen, stimulating hormonal balance, and flushing out the muscles, organs and lymphatic system."

Physically, beyond improving muscle tone, strength and stamina, yoga boosts metabolism, which aids in weight loss. It also increases joint range of motion, making you less prone to injury. Yoga is internally therapeutic too: whether you're hoping to improve digestion or stimulate the thyroid, there's likely a pose to counteract your ailment, as well as support your organs, muscles, joints and vessels. For instance, the Triangle Pose improves circulation, while the Bridge relieves menstrual and menopausal discomfort.

Yoga is mentally and emotionally restorative too. Feeling frazzled? Improve your focus with Warrior III. Stifled? Liberate yourself with the Fish Pose. From muscular to skeletal, reproductive to endocrine, nervous to glandular, on a physical and physiological level, yoga balances all our systems.

## Issues Treated by Yoga Therapy

Yoga therapy is a growing field and scientific evidence has begun to emphasize its efficacy. It is used to treat existing mental and physical health issues, but can also be used as a self-care strategy for prevention and maintenance.

Yoga therapy is well established as a treatment for depression and anxiety. A meta-analysis cited in the Primary Care Companion for CNS Disorders found that it also shows promise in the treatment of post-traumatic stress disorder (PTSD) and schizophrenia. Yoga therapists have also begun to develop treatment modalities to suit children with autism. The book *Yoga Therapy for Children with Autism and Special Needs*, written in 2013 by yoga teacher Louise Goldberg, is already considered a critical text for novice and experienced yoga therapists alike.

According to a 2012 article in *Social Work Today* magazine, yoga therapy is also emerging as an effective treatment for substance abuse issues. Mental health professionals point out that yoga positively affects the parts of the mind and body susceptible to addiction. Studies have shown that yoga boosts the neurotransmitter GABA (gamma-aminobutyric acid), which is important because GABA levels are statistically low in people who experience substance abuse, anxiety and depression.

Because of its concentration on mind and body integration, yoga therapy is also used to address many physical health issues. It has been effectively used to treat back pain, heart conditions, asthma, chronic fatigue, hypertension, multiple sclerosis and side effects of chemotherapy.

## Practice and Benefits of Yoga Therapy

Yoga therapy is practiced in a wide range of formats. Physical therapists, for example, often implement yoga techniques in massage and other treatments. Yoga therapy practice can resemble physical therapy, rehabilitative therapy and/or psychotherapy. Unlike a standard yoga class, yoga therapy sessions are typically conducted in one-on-one or small group settings. Yoga therapy can be provided as an adjunct to complement other forms of treatment or can be used to directly treat a specific issue. Yoga techniques range from simple to advanced and can be enjoyed by people of all ages. Potential benefits from yoga therapy include stress reduction, psychological well-being, improved diet and efficient functioning of bodily systems.

## History of Yoga Therapy

Yoga therapy is rooted in the ancient practice of yoga, which originated thousands of years ago in India. Yoga made its way to the United States in the late 1800s, but yoga therapy formally emerged in the 1980s as the result of a study conducted by Dr Dean Ornish. It illustrated how the implementation of a healthy lifestyle program could reverse heart disease. Ornish's program included therapeutic yoga and was the first to highlight the benefits of using yoga in this way. This program for treating heart disease was approved for insurance coverage in 1990 and it marked the beginning of the medical field's acceptance of yoga as a treatment option.

In 1983, the Biomedical Yoga Trust was founded to further develop and standardize yoga therapy. The International Association of Yoga Therapists (IAYT) was founded in 1989 and has since hosted yoga conferences, published the Journal of the International Association of Yoga Therapists and contributed to creating yoga therapy training standards. Both organizations have facilitated research to explore the extent of yoga therapy's potential.

## What to Expect from Yoga Therapy?

When a person decides to initiate yoga therapy, the therapist will first conduct an initial assessment. This is designed to do the following:

- Identify health problems
- Assess lifestyle and physical capability
- Discuss reasons for seeking therapy
- Create a course of treatment

Once the treatment plan is established in this first consultation, the frequency of sessions is agreed upon and sessions are scheduled. From this point, therapy sessions will most likely include the following:

Breathing Exercises (Pranayama): The therapist will guide the person in therapy through a series of breathing exercises ranging from energizing to balancing breaths.

Physical Postures (Asana): The therapist will teach the person in treatment appropriate yoga poses that address problem areas. For example, the "Legs Up the Wall" pose is used to treat things like anxiety and insomnia. In this pose, the person lays on his or her back with legs positioned up against the wall.

Meditation: Relaxation and mindfulness are the focus of meditation when it is combined with yoga poses.

Guided Imagery: The yoga therapist needs to calm the body and mind by providing a guided visualization intended to bring inner peace.

Homework: An important element for any yoga practice is to find a way to incorporate it into daily life. Yoga therapists should provide instructions on how to use what has been learned in treatment at home.

## Panchakosha, the Five Layers of Existence

**Taittriya Upanishad** explains the concept of **Pancha Kosha**, the five layers of existence.

**Annamaya Kosha:** It is the physical body or the gross body. The physical body is made up of Pancha Bhutas, the five elements, namely Prithivi or earth, Apa or water, Tejas or fire, Vayu or wind and Akasha or space. This is normally nourished by the food we consume. Hence, the statement "you are what you eat."

**Pranamaya Kosha:** It is the pranic or subtle body. Prāna is the basic fabric of life. A harmonious flow of prāna to every cell of the body keeps them alive and healthy. Prāna has the capacity to move into different areas of the body depending on demand. For example, when you perform tasks that engage the brain, you need more prāna in the head. When you walk, you need more prāna in the lower limbs. When there is disturbance in this prāna, it leads to dysfunction in the physical body.

**Manomaya Kosha:** It is the mind body. Mind is defined as the conglomeration of thoughts. When a thought circulates in the mind and chitta, it soon goes on to make you feel "I want it." This component of Manomaya Kosha is called Emotion or Bhavana. This is characterized by feelings such as "likes or dislikes," "love or hate," baked by the "I," the ego. It is this emotion that is the root cause of all human joy and distress. The imbalance in this sheath is known as "Adhi" or stress. Long-standing Adhis get pushed into Pranamaya Kosha and Annamaya Kosha causing Vyadis. Manomaya Kosha is our mental and emotional library, the subtler layer of our existence. Hence the statement "you are what you think."

**Vignanamaya Kosha:** This is the intellectual body. The conscience within that continuously guides us to do or not to do something is the Vignanamaya Kosha. It is this component of the mind that has developed considerably among humans, differentiating them from animals. Hunger, sleep, fear and the procreative instinct are common to man and animals. It is Buddhi, the discrimination faculty, which is special to man. A person who does not have Buddhi is equal to an animal.

**Anandamaya Kosha:** It is the Bliss body. Anandamaya Kosha is the Bliss layer of our existence. This is the subtlest aspect of our existence, a state of complete harmony and perfect health. Reaching this state is the ultimate goal of any human being.

## Science of Illness (Vyadhi)

Vyadhi are of two types: Adhija Vyadhi and Anadhija Vyadhi.

**Adhija Vyadhi:** All stress-related diseases are Adhija Vyadhis. Adhi starts at Manomaya Kosha and percolates into the Pranamaya Kosha and then Annamaya Kosha and results in a disease. Stress is of two types: Sara—essential stress and Samanya—ordinary stress.

**Anadhija Vyadhi:** This refers to diseases that are not stress-related. These mainly include accidents, infectious and contagious diseases.

We can manage this wide category of diseases effectively through yoga.

## Yoga Practice for Specific Goals

Yoga practice is for several goals like:

- Improving posture
- Enhancing body awareness
- Increasing strength
- Increasing joint freedom and flexibility

- Cardiovascular fitness
- Digestive health
- Relief from pain
- Managing stress
- Strengthening the immune system
- Meditation training to develop a spiritual practice
- Using yoga as a therapy

# 77 Surprising Health Benefits of Yoga

Over the past several years, yoga has experienced an upsurge in popularity in the Western world among medical professionals and celebrities alike. While many associate yoga with new-age mysticism or the latest fad at the gym, yoga is an ancient practice that connects the mind, body and spirit through body poses, controlled breathing and meditation. The practice of yoga has many health benefits associated with it, so read below to discover 77 benefits of incorporating yoga into your or your patient's fitness program.

## *Wellness Benefits*

From lowering blood pressure to increasing pain tolerance, the following health benefits can all be discovered within the body.

1. **Blood pressure.** Consistent yoga practice decreases blood pressure through better circulation and oxygenation of the body.
2. **Pulse rate.** A slower pulse rate indicates that your heart is strong enough to pump more blood with fewer beats. Regular yoga practice provides a lower pulse rate.
3. **Circulation.** Yoga improves blood circulation. By transporting nutrients and oxygen throughout your body, yoga practice provides healthier organs, skin and brain.
4. **Respiration.** Like the circulatory system, a lower respiratory rate indicates that the lungs are working more efficiently. Yoga decreases the respiratory rate through a combination of controlled breathing exercises and better fitness.
5. **Cardiovascular endurance.** A combination of lower heart rate and improved oxygenation to the body (both benefits of yoga) results in higher cardiovascular endurance.
6. **Organs.** Yoga practice massages internal organs, thus improving the body's ability to prevent disease. An experienced yoga practitioner also becomes better attuned to her body, being able to quickly detect if something isn't functioning properly, thereby allowing for quicker response to head off disease.
7. **Gastrointestinal.** Gastrointestinal functions have been shown to improve in both men and women who practice yoga.
8. **Immunity.** Yoga practice has frequently been correlated with a stronger immune system, including some poses that specifically work on areas of immunity.

9. **Pain**. Pain tolerance is much higher among those who practice yoga regularly. In addition to pain tolerance, some instances of chronic pain, such as back pain, are lessened or eliminated through yoga.

10. **Metabolism**. Having a balanced metabolism helps maintain a healthy weight and control hunger. Consistent yoga practice helps find the balance and creates a more efficient metabolism.

## *Physical Health Benefits*

Just as many health benefits occur within the body, there are many benefits that can be experienced externally. From better sleep to more energy and strength, yoga has several benefits.

1. **Aging**. Yoga stimulates the detoxification process within the body. Detoxification has been shown to delay aging, among many other health benefits.

2. **Posture**. The very nature of yoga teaches the practitioner how to hold and control one's body in a more healthful position. Through consistent practice, your posture will improve so that you look more confident and healthy.

3. **Strength**. One of the premises of yoga is that you are using the weight of your own body for overall strength.

4. **Energy**. Regular yoga practice provides consistent energy. In fact, most yogis state that when you perform yoga correctly, you will feel energized after your yoga session rather than tired.

5. **Weight**. The benefits of better metabolism along with the exercise of yoga keep your weight in check. Additionally, the stretching of muscles helps to reduce the amount of cellulite that can build around muscles.

6. **Sleep**. Because of yoga's many benefits to both body and mind, many find that their sleep is much better.

7. **Balance**. An integral part of yoga practice is balance and control over your body. With consistent practice, you will find that your overall balance will improve outside the yoga class.

8. **Integrated function of the body**. Yoga is derived from Sanskrit and means "to join together and direct one's attention." This is exactly what happens to your body after you start practicing yoga. Yogis find that their body works together much better, resulting in more graceful and efficient body movements.

9. **Body awareness**: Doing yoga will give you an increased awareness of your own body. You are often called upon to make small, subtle movements to improve your alignment. Over time, this will increase your level of comfort in your own body. This can lead to improved posture and greater self-confidence.

10. **Core strength**. With a strong body core, you achieve better posture and overall body strength. A strong core helps heal and reduce injuries. This is why a lot of athletes do yoga as cross training.

11. **Sexuality**. Yoga can improve your sexuality through better control, more relaxation and more self-confidence.

## *Emotional Health Benefits*

Due to the strong mind-body connection of yoga, there are many emotional benefits to be gained from consistent yoga practice.

1.  **Mood**. Overall well-being improves with yoga practice. The combination of creating a strong mind-body connection, a healthy body and focusing inward can lead to improvement in your mood.

2.  **Stress reduction**. The concentration required during yoga practice tends to focus your attention on the matter at hand, thereby reducing the emphasis you may have been putting on the stress in your life.

3.  **Anxiety**. One benefit of the controlled breathing used in yoga is a reduction in anxiety.

4.  **Depression**. Some believe the negative feelings that you may be repressing are brought to the surface during some types of yoga exercise. When this happens, negative energy is no longer stuck within you, but released through exercise. Regularly releasing this negativity leads to a reduction of depression in many people.

5.  **Self-acceptance**. Focusing inward and realizing through your yoga practice that perfection is not the goal allows for self-acceptance.

6.  **Self-control**. The controlled movements of yoga teach you how to translate that self-control to all aspects of your life.

7.  **Mind-body connection**. Few other exercises offer the same mind-body connection that yoga does. As you match your controlled breathing with the movements of your body, you retrain your mind to find that place of calm and peace that long-time yogis know.

8.  **Positive outlook on life**. Continued practice of yoga results in a balance of many hormones and the nervous system, which brings about a more stable, positive approach to life.

9.  **Hostility**. Most yogis report a huge reduction in the amount of hostility they feel as well as a sense of control when anger flares. This calm effect is likely from the relaxation and meditation that is incorporated in their yoga practice, leading to an overall calming of the nervous system. Less hostility means lower blood pressure and stress and a healthier approach to life.

10.  **Concentration**. Researchers have shown that as little as 8 weeks of yoga practice can result in better concentration and more motivation.

11.  **Memory**. Improved blood circulation to the brain as well as reduction in stress and improved focus results in a better memory.

12.  **Attention**. The attention required in yoga to maintain the structured breathing in conjunction with yoga poses sharpens the ability to keep a sharp focus on tasks.

13.  **Social skills**. In yoga, you learn the interconnectedness of all of life. Your yoga practice soon evolves from a personal journey to one connecting to the community at large where your social skills improve along with your yoga practice.

14. **Calmness**. Concentrating so intently on what your body is doing brings calmness. Yoga also introduces you to meditation techniques, such as watching how you breathe and disengaging from your thoughts, which help calm the mind.

## Body Chemistry Benefits

Several aspects of body chemistry such as glucose levels and red blood cells are affected by yoga.

1. **Cholesterol**. Yoga practice lowers cholesterol by increasing blood circulation and burning fat. Yoga practice is a great tool to fight harmful cholesterol levels.

2. **Lymphatic system**. Your lymphatic system boosts your immunity and reduces toxins in your body. The only way to get it working well is by movement. The specific movements involved in yoga are particularly well-suited for promoting a strong lymphatic system.

3. **Glucose**. There is evidence to suggest that yoga may lower blood glucose levels.

4. **Sodium**. Like any good exercise program, yoga reduces the sodium levels in your body. In today's world of processed and fast foods that are full of sodium, lessening these levels is a great idea.

5. **Endocrine functions**. Practicing yoga helps regulate and control hormone secretion. An improved endocrine system keeps hormones in balance and promotes better physical and emotional health.

6. **Triglycerides**. Triglycerides are the chemical form of fat in blood, and elevated levels can indicate a risk of heart disease and high blood pressure. A recent study shows that yoga can lead to "significantly lower" levels of triglycerides.

7. **Red blood cells**. Yoga has been shown to increase the level of red blood cells in the body. Red blood cells are responsible for carrying oxygen through the blood, and too few can result in anemia and low energy.

8. **Vitamin C**. Vitamin C helps boost immunity, produce collagen and is a powerful antioxidant. A yoga regimen can increase the Vitamin C in your body.

## Exercise Benefits

As a form of exercise, yoga offers benefits that are sometimes not easily found among other exercise regimens.

1. **Low risk of injury**. Due to the low impact of yoga and the controlled aspect of the motions, the risk of injury during yoga practice is very low compared to other forms of exercise.

2. **Parasympathetic nervous system**. In many forms of exercise, the sympathetic nervous system kicks in, providing you with that fight-or-flight sensation. Yoga does the opposite and stimulates the parasympathetic nervous system, which lowers blood pressure and slows your breathing, allowing relaxation and healing.

3. **Muscle tone**. Consistently practicing yoga leads to better muscle tone.

4. **Sub-cortex**. Subcortical regions of the brain are associated with well-being, and yoga is thought to dominate the sub-cortex rather than the cortex (where most exercise dominates).

5. **Reduced oxygen consumption**. Yoga consumes less oxygen than traditional exercise routines, thereby allowing the body to work more efficiently.

6. **Breathing**. With yoga, breathing is more natural and controlled during exercise. This provides more oxygen-rich air for your body and more energy with less fatigue.

7. **Balanced workout of opposing muscle groups**. As with all of yoga, balance is key. If a muscle group is worked in one direction, it will also be worked in the opposite direction to maintain balance. This results in a better overall workout for the body.

8. **Non-competitive**. The introspective and self-building nature of yoga removes any need for competition in the exercise regimen. With the lack of competition, the yogi is free to work slowly to avoid any undue injury and promote a more balanced and stress-free workout.

9. **Joint range of motion**. A study at the University of Pennsylvania School of Medicine indicated that joint range of motion was improved by participants who practiced yoga.

10. **Eye-hand coordination**. Without practice, eye-hand coordination diminishes. Yoga maintains and improves eye-hand coordination.

11. **Dexterity**. The strong mind-body connection and flexibility gained from yoga leads to grace and skill.

12. **Reaction time**. Research done in India shows that reaction time can be improved with specific yoga breathing exercises in conjunction with an already established yoga practice. The improvement was attributed to the faster rate of processing and improved concentration gained from yoga.

13. **Endurance**. Working the entire body, yoga improves endurance and is frequently used by endurance athletes as a supplement to their sport-specific training.

14. **Depth perception**. Becoming aware of your body and how it moves, as one does in yoga practice, leads to increased depth perception.

## Disease Prevention

Doctors and nurses love yoga because studies indicate that it can help prevent the following diseases.

1. **Heart disease**. Yoga reduces stress, lowers blood pressure, keeps off weight and improves cardiovascular health, all of which reduce your risk of heart disease.

2. **Osteoporosis**. It is well documented that weight-bearing exercise strengthens bones and helps prevent osteoporosis. Additionally, yoga's ability to lower levels of cortisol may help keep calcium in the bones.

3. **Alzheimer's**. A new study indicates that yoga can help raise brain gamma-aminobutyric (GABA) levels. Low GABA levels are associated with the onset of Alzheimer's. Meditation as practiced in yoga has also been shown to slow the progression of Alzheimer's.

4. **Type II diabetes**. Yoga reduces glucose, is an excellent source of physical exercise and stress reduction and can potentially encourage insulin production, all of which can help prevent type II diabetes.

## *Symptom Reduction or Alleviation*

Medical professionals have learned that the following diseases or disorders can all be helped through the practice of yoga.

1. **Carpal tunnel syndrome.** Individuals with carpal tunnel syndrome who practiced yoga showed greater improvement than those who wore a splint or received no treatment at all. Researchers saw improved grip strength and reduction of pain in study participants.

2. **Asthma.** Evidence suggests that reducing symptoms of asthma and even reduction in asthma medication are the result of regular yoga.

3. **Arthritis.** The slow, deliberate movement of yoga poses coupled with the gentle pressure exerted on joints is excellent in relieving arthritis symptoms. Also, the stress relief associated with yoga loosens muscles that tighten joints.

4. **Multiple sclerosis.** Yoga is now recognized as an excellent means of multiple sclerosis management.

5. **Cancer.** Those fighting or recovering from cancer frequently take advantage of the benefits that yoga provides. Cancer patients who practice yoga gain strength, raise red blood cells, experience less nausea during chemotherapy and have better overall well-being.

6. **Muscular dystrophy.** Using yoga in the early stages of muscular dystrophy can help return some physical functions. The practice of Pranayam yoga helped one teen regain many of his abilities lost to muscular dystrophy.

7. **Migraines.** Regular yoga practice has been shown to reduce the number of migraines in chronic migraine sufferers.

8. **Scoliosis.** Yoga can straighten the spine curvature associated with scoliosis.

9. **Chronic bronchitis.** Exercise that does not elevate respiration yet increases oxygen levels is ideal for treating chronic bronchitis. Luckily, yoga can do this, as well as aerate the lungs and provide energy.

10. **Epilepsy.** By focusing on stress reduction, breathing and restoring overall balance in the body yoga can help prevent epileptic seizures.

11. **Sciatica.** The intense pain associated with sciatica can be alleviated with specific yoga poses.

12. **Obsessive Compulsive Disorder.** Studies of people with obsessive compulsive disorder have shown that practicing yoga led to a reduction in symptoms, resulting in less medication or even doing away with the need for medication.

13. **Constipation.** Due to the practice of yoga and overall better posture, the digestive and elimination systems work more efficiently. If the practitioner also has a healthy diet, constipation will be eliminated through yoga.

14. **Allergies.** Using a neti pot to clear the sinuses is an ancient form of yoga to help reduce or eliminate allergy symptoms. Certain types of breathing can also help clear the nasal passages.

15. **Menopause.** Yoga practice can help control some of the side effects of menopause.

16. **Back pain.** Yoga reduces spinal compression and helps overall body alignment to reduce back pain.

# 40 Ways Yoga Heals

1. Increases flexibility
2. Strengthens muscles
3. Improves balance
4. Improves immune function
5. Improves posture
6. Improves lung capacity
7. Leads to lower and deeper breathing
8. Discourages mouth breathing
9. Increases oxygenation of tissues
10. Improves joint health
11. Nourishes inter-vertebral discs
12. Improves return of venous blood
13. Increases function of the feet
14. Increases circulation of lymph
15. Improves proprioception
16. Increases control of bodily functions
17. Strengthens bones
18. Conditions the cardiovascular system
19. Promotes weight loss
20. Relaxes the nervous system
21. Improves the function of the nervous system
22. Improves brain function
23. Activates the left prefrontal cortex
24. Changes neurotransmitter levels
25. Lowers levels of the stress hormone cortisol
26. Lowers blood sugar
27. Lowers blood pressure
28. Improves levels of cholesterol and triglycerides
29. Thins the blood
30. Improves bowel function
31. Releases unconscious muscular gripping
32. Uses imagery to effect change in the body
33. Relieves pain
34. Lowers need for medication
35. Fosters healing relationship

36. Improves psychological health

37. Leads to healthier habits

38. Fosters spiritual growth

39. Elicits the placebo effect

40. Encourages involvement in our own healing

# Improving Posture

To perfect your posture and poise, the following muscles (refer to the diagram on muscular system in Chapter 1 to locate these muscles) need to be strengthened regularly:

- The psoas, which supports the spine and balances the pelvic girdle upon the thighs.
- The gluteus maximus, which is responsible for the power of the pelvis and legs and supports the spinal column at the lumbar region.
- The latissimus dorsi, which makes up two-thirds of the back.
- The erector spinae, which with the latissimus dorsi keeps the trunk erect.
- The trapezius, which opens the chest and maintains neck and shoulder posture.
- The rectus abdominis is antagonistic to the psoas. They need to work harmoniously to maintain the posture of the abdominal and lower back regions.

If these muscles are regularly exercised, your posture will improve. Postural strength is greatly enhanced by understanding how these muscles work and learning to utilize them in daily movements. Specific postural imbalances can be improved by following the recommendations in the table below. The individual poses of your customized routine should be progressively developed for up to 12 breaths each to maximize your stamina.

## Yoga Therapy Recommendations for Postural Imbalances

| Postural Change | Therapeutic Yogasanas |
|---|---|
| Body leans forward | Hero, Energy Freeing, Camel |
| Body leans backward | Extended Triangle, Downward-Facing Dog, Squat |
| Forward head | Cobra, Extended Triangle, Camel |
| Tilted head | Extended Triangle, Abdominal Twist, Spinal Twist |
| High shoulder | Same as above; adjust scapula downward, contracting lower trapezius, latissimus |
| Round shoulders | Warrior I, Downward-Facing Dog, Camel |
| Arm turned out | Upward Extended Legs, Stick, Westside Back Stretch |
| Arm turned in | Bridge, Spinal Twist, Camel |
| Arm out from hip | Stick, Camel, Bound Angle |
| Winging scapula | Bridge, Supported Shoulder Stand, Cobra |
| Flat back | Side-of-Hip Stretch, Head-to-Knee, Back Stretch |

| Postural Change | Therapeutic Yogasanas |
|---|---|
| Lordosis (excessive lumbar curve) | Upward Legs, Boat, Reclining Hero |
| Scoliosis (lateral curve) | Side-of-Hip Stretch, Extended Triangle, Head-to-Knee |
| Khyphosis (hunchback) | Downward-Facing Dog, Bridge, Camel |
| High hip | Side-of-Hip Stretch, Head-to-Knee, Half Locust |
| Hip twisted | Warrior I, Abdominal Twist, Spinal Twist |
| Hyperextended knee | Warrior II, Bridge, Camel |
| Knock-knees | Balancing Tree, Warrior II, Head to Knee Bowed Legs Warrior I, Side-of-Hip Stretch, Face of Light Leg Outward Warrior I, Side-of-Hip Stretch, Boat |
| Leg inward | Balancing Tree, Extended Triangle, Face of Light |
| Fallen arch/Flat foot | Mountain (balance on toes), Hero, Fetal |

## Chapter 7

# MEDITATION AND RELAXATION

"We are taught how to move and behave in the external world, but we are never taught how to be still and examine what is within ourselves. At the same time, learning to be still and calm should not be made ceremony or a part of any religion; it is a universal requirement of the human body. When one learns to sit still, he or she attains a kind of joy that is inexplicable. The highest of all joys that can ever be attained or experienced by a human being can be attained through meditation. All the other joys in the world are transient and momentary, but the joy of meditation is immense and everlasting," says Swami Rama, in *Meditation and its Practice*.

Meditation will take us to a state of awareness of our true being, a state of complete and spontaneous relaxation, innocence and bliss. Initially, most of us have trouble focusing the mind and keeping it positive, but the sages urge and advise us to stay focused so that meditation becomes an integral part of everyday life, as basic and necessary as eating and sleeping. By definition, meditation is transcendental, in which all fears, desires, longings, negative emotions and even positive attachment are left behind.

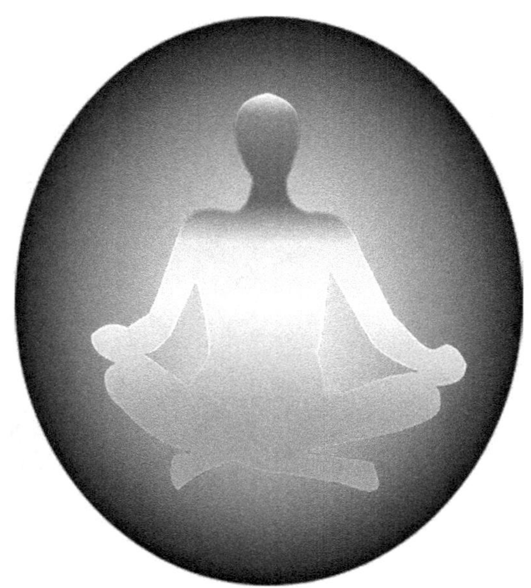

Meditation teaches about the power within each of us: the energy, peace and wisdom, we can tap into once we know it is available. Many different names and forms exist for this inner power such as Cosmic Consciousness, Holy Spirit, Universal Mind, Love, the Peace that Passes all Understanding, the Absolute; others call it Buddha, Christ, Allah, Brahmin and God. Although the paths are many, only one supreme essence exists and pervades all life.

Understanding, defining and describing this limitless and boundless Self is impossible. Only through the practice of meditation and direct experience can this essence be known. Through meditation we can also still the mind, develop intuitive abilities and touch the supreme essence, achieving peace, compassion, joy and understanding in the process.

Yoga differs from Western philosophical teachings since it focuses on the Self only and not on others. Yoga teaches that to find peace we must first develop peace within ourselves. The challenge is to gain control of our own internal world. In a constantly moving and changing world, meditation teaches us to slow down and focus the mind.

Meditation is a state of consciousness, a steady flow of uninterrupted consciousness; it is not a void but the fullness of pure consciousness itself. While stilling the mind, we fruitlessly find selfless love, the very source of bliss. Through misguided actions and thought patterns, we have mislaid this natural state. To find our true nature, we need to realign ourselves to the eternal, universal laws of health, love and harmony. These are the optimal conditions needed to practice the art of meditation. The journey to a quiet mind, away from unhealthy and unrewarding states, is a long and challenging one. This journey requires patience, perseverance and tenacity, but is a promising one filled with joy, awareness and deeper meaning.

## Yoga Therapy Recommendations for Postural Imbalances

Meditation is a process and, as such, takes time. A degree of willpower is needed to remain in the state of heightened awareness, but at the same time, you need to relax, letting go of all expectations and desires. The art of meditation lies in the balance between the efforts needed to sustain concentration and the detachment from all distractions.

### 1. The Place

Maintain a space to be used solely for meditation, clean, tidy and free from distracting vibrations. Keep it sacred to you, a place of focus. Set up a table in the room with a light source (candle, oil lamp) which is a potent spiritual symbol. Your sacred space will soon have a magnetic aura created by you during meditation. In times of stress you can retreat to your space, practice and experience comfort and relief. Purify your meditation area of negative energy using a short ritual called arati at the end of each meditation session. In this ceremony, a flame is offered in your place of meditation while mantras (chanting) are repeated. While traveling, arati will help purify your new area of meditation, clearing negative energies. Arati will help strengthen the energy changes brought on in meditation within and around you.

Direction: by turning your table to the North or East, you will take full advantage of favorable magnetic vibrations. Meditating in nature will do away with the distractions of meditating in the city: noise, pollution, machinery and high stress levels. Take advantage of any opportunity to meditate in nature.

## 2. The Time

The most favorable and effective time to practice meditation is at dawn and dusk. The most desirable time is in between 4 and 6 am, called Brahmamuhurta. In these hours, the mind and atmosphere are clean and unruffled by activities of the day. Around sunset and just before bed are also good times. No matter what time is favorable for you, make sure that you will not be disturbed by outside distractions.

## 3. The Habit

Consistency in meditation is important. Try to meditate at the same time every day. Start with 15 minutes and work your way up to an hour. It is important to practice every day. Soon, you will crave meditation and you will not feel full without it.

## 4. The Sitting Position

Sit in a comfortable position with a relaxed but erect spine and neck. The psychic current needs to travel unimpeded from the base of the spine to the top of the head, helping to steady the mind and encourage concentration. Sitting in Padmasana (Classic Full Lotus), Siddhasana (Half Lotus) or in Sukhasana (Simple Cross-legged Pose) provides a triangular flow of energy, containing it rather than allowing it to disperse in all directions. The mild muscular contraction necessary to hold the back upright in a sitting position keeps you alert. Try to relax the rest of your body as much as possible. You can place your hands on your knees in the chin-mudra position with your forefinger and thumb touching. The positions should be pleasant but firm (says Patanjali), and one should feel as steady as a mountain outwardly and as flowing as honey within (says Swami Sivananda).

## 5. The Breath

Consciously try to breathe rhythmically. Begin with deep abdominal breathing and move to a slower rate. Inhale and exhale rhythmically for approximately three seconds each.

## 6. The Mind

For your meditation practice to succeed, it is important to transform your suffering and negativity by welcoming heightened awareness, broad vision, joy and contentment into your life. Commit to living in the present; give up living in the past and daydreaming or worrying about the future. Meditation allows us to see things as they are, without the masking veil of our likes and dislikes, fear or hope. Detachment from all hopes and fears protects against suffering. Your life will be greatly enhanced by gently commanding the mind to be quiet for a specific length of time and by focusing only on the present moment.

## 7. Choosing a Point of Concentration

To anchor the mind, start by bringing awareness to the posture and breath. Further the strength of concentration by bringing all your attention to a specific point in the body. These points are called chakras or energy centers. Seven major chakras exist in the body and there are many more secondary ones. They are located in the astral body (body of energy) along the spinal column. The chakras correspond to different levels of consciousness or to the different levels of expressions of our inner energies. The three lower chakras correspond to the basic desires of the mind: security, pleasure and expression of individuality. The fourth (heart) chakra corresponds to the expression of our energy as love. The fifth (throat) chakra is the center where consciousness expands to encompass knowledge of past and future incarnations. The sixth chakra, between the eyebrows, is the center for intuitional knowledge. The last chakra, on top of the head, corresponds to a state of union with cosmic consciousness. Swami Sivananda suggests that when meditating, we should focus on either the heart center (anahata chakra), being more emotional, loving and nurturing in nature or the center between the eyebrows (ajna chakra), being more logical, analytical and intellectual. Using the ajna chakra will uplift the intellect, open the doors of intuition and let you perceive reality without the limited screen of intellect. This state is referred to as the opening of the third eye. Remember that once you have chosen a point of concentration, keep it for the rest of your life. Focusing on your point is a springboard for concentration, but try not to confine the mind while focusing. Meditation is not merely an act of will, but more a commitment of the heart. Where your heart goes, your mind goes; where your mind goes, your life will follow.

## 8. Choosing an Object of Concentration

All previous steps are a preparation for this step. Mantras are an essential tool for concentration. You can start the practice by repeating the mantra aloud. Gradually, lower your voice to a whisper and then reduce it to the most powerful method, mental repetition. A mantra is a powerful tool, channeling two aspects of the mind: the desires to see and to hear. You can also repeat a mantra and visualize any symbol of an uplifting or agreeable nature. The symbol, from the Om to the Christian cross, should have the inherent power to take your mind to the infinite.

## 9. Giving Space to the Mind

At first, let your mind wander a bit and then settle slowly. Be patient with yourself and focus gently. Change must happen consciously, progressively and steadily to have a lasting effect. Both love and strength are necessary when educating your mind. Remember to avoid overindulgence and harshness; realize that your accomplishments, no matter how small, are something to be proud of. During the first few minutes of your practice, develop a relationship of trust with your mind by being patient and compassionate. As the *Bhagavad Gita* says, become your own best friend and feel compassion for the part of you that is struggling to regain a sense of wholeness.

## 10. Disassociating from the Mind

When the mind persists in wandering, disassociate from it and watch it objectively as an impartial witness, as though you were watching a film. At first you may be discouraged so try the attitude of non-cooperation. Know that you are not the mind, but only a spectator. If you stop interacting, entertaining and feeding your emotions and thoughts with consciousness, then they will simply have no energy to live and will lose strength and intensity. With practice, your mind will gradually slow down.

## 11. Pure Thought

Pure thought means no thought. Sustained concentration leads to meditation, but this may take months and years of practice.

## 12. SamāDhi, the Highest State of Meditation

Sustained meditation leads to Samādhi. Here, duality disappears and you enter the super conscious state: the state of peace, joy, love, equanimity and contentment. Change does occur to those who meditate regularly, but do not set up expectations for change because you may become discouraged when they do not occur in the timely fashion you anticipated. There are universal indicators that all who meditate will experience sooner or later.

### Meditation, a Great Energizer

Meditation is a vigorous tonic to the physical system. Although previously skeptical, scientists now believe the mind can control the activity of a single cell as well as a group of cells. When thoughts and desires pour into the body, the cells are activated and the body obeys the group demand. The powerful soothing ways of prana penetrate the cells and exercise a benign influence on all organs, setting in motion the healing and strengthening that prevents and cures many diseases.

Meditation helps to prolong the body's anabolic process of cell production, growth and repair and reduce the anabolic process of decay. Once you practice meditation regularly, sleep can be reduced with no fatigue, you will develop a powerful digestive system and your senses will sharpen, resulting in heightened perception.

Meditation is a great energizer and will make you feel and look healthier.

Achieving calmness of mind: Real progress in your practice is accurately measured in the waking state. By observing yourself without judgment or praise you will lessen the control of your habitual thoughts and emotions. Negative tendencies will decrease and your mind will become steadier; your face will be calm and serene.

Development of inner clarity: The practice of concentration increases willpower and memory, resulting in a sharp and bright intellect. You will have a one-pointed, clear, strong, subtle mind with clear-cut mental images and well-defined and well-grounded thoughts. You will discriminate and detach from the drama of day-to-day living, resulting in less stress and more peace.

Gradual transformation of personality: This new-found peace will change your lifestyle and universal views. Lethargy and laziness disappear as cheerfulness and joy grows. You will live in the present and start to live simply and without clutter. As you advance in your practice you will gradually develop a love for all. You will find that you are less affected by daily turmoil, keeping a cool head and a balanced mind. You will develop a magnetic and dynamic personality; you will attract people to you and lift their moods and minds.

Remember that progress will not manifest immediately and it may take years before you start to reap the most profound benefits. Stay focused and motivated and have no expectations. You will see changes and improvements in your life at all levels. It is very important to not become complacent and curtail your practice. Do not become self-satisfied because the mind's layers of impurities run deep and it is only when you start to work on them that you realize how many there are. Great patience, perseverance, vigilance and undaunted strength are needed. Be firm, steady and steadfast. You will engage in rich and rewarding relationships as you learn to understand yourself and others better; you will experience a full and well-lived life as you take control in ways that previously seemed impossible. Meditation paves the way for perfection; continue your practice and reap the beauty of peace and stillness that will slowly unfold.

## Challenges to Meditation

The work of changing behavior and personality may be difficult, but see each hurdle as a test to strengthen the mind. The mind increases in power when it overcomes challenges. When you sit for meditation, it is common for negative thoughts to flood into the mind. Do not forcibly get rid of these thoughts because they will turn against your will and then double the energy. Instead, return to your mantra and know that conscious uneasiness due to negative thoughts is already a step forward.

- Sleep: Drowsiness and sleep are common obstacles in the practice of meditation. Through yogic practices, you develop a calm and steady mind, become more relaxed and consequently, need less sleep. Sometimes during meditation practice, you may be unsure whether you have slipped into sleep or not. If you have or if sleeping becomes a problem during meditation, splash cold water on your face, do breathing exercises or stand on your head for five minutes.

- Lethargy: Lethargy and depression often affect the beginner. Take care of your health and well-being with regular exercise and a healthy diet and avoid tedious mental work, too much or too little sleep and excessive sexual activity. Bring rhythm into your life by establishing a daily routine of meditation, exercise and study. Cheerfulness goes hand-in-hand with health.

- Too much talking: Excessive talking diminishes spiritual power and hinders the practice of meditation. The wise speak few words and only when necessary. To help calm, center and discipline the mind, try to practice mouna or silence, for up to an hour each day, over and above the time spent mediating. Resisting the temptation to join in conversation or discussion at every opportunity can be regarded as a form of mouna. The traits of self-justification, self-assertion, obstinacy, dissimulation and lying are associated with talking too much. If you readily admit faults, mistakes and weaknesses, then your mind will start to calm and meditation will become easier.

- Negative influences: This includes anybody or anything that pulls the mind away from peacefulness. If possible, try to avoid people who lie, steal, are greedy or indulge in criticism and gossip. Try to associate with those whose inspirations are uplifting and inspiring.

- Discouragement: After a while, doubts may arise about the effectiveness of practicing meditation. Remember that there are always periods when progress seems a little slow. Conversing with people of strong faith and firm practice clears all doubts. Continue to practice with no regard for the outcome. Growth will come, but it is always gradual. Sincerity, regularity and patience will bring progress.

- Anger: Anger is the most devastating barrier to mediation and the greatest enemy of peace. It gains strength with repetition and is difficult to control once it becomes habitual. When you control anger, all other shortcomings die by themselves and the will gradually strengthens. When you are irritated, practice patience immediately, speak moderately and if anger rises, stop speaking and turn your attention elsewhere. Drink cool water or take a brisk walk to help calm yourself.

- Smoking, eating meat and drinking alcohol: These increase rājas, which aggravates the mind; they are best avoided.

- Fear: It is debilitating and will severely hamper your ability to meditate. Fear of public criticism especially can stand in the way of your meditation progress. Friends, colleagues and even close family may mock or criticize you for your practice. Hold on to your practice, even in the face of ridicule.

- Hatred: This is a great obstacle to the mind of a serious practitioner. Hatred creates more hatred. Contempt, prejudice and ridicule are some of the most damaging forms hatred takes. You can have your own principles and your own standards and modes of behaviors and still respect the viewpoints and actions of others. Truth is not the sole monopoly of any person, group or spiritual system. Gossiping, criticizing and being judgmental are some of the subtler manifestations of hatred. Peace of mind and universal peace is only possible when hatred, prejudice and bigotry have been replaced with love.

- Dwelling in the past: When you sit for meditation, vivid thoughts of past experiences may appear. Dreams of your childhood, schooldays and youth are just dreams and should be laid gently but permanently to rest. Try to let go of all the thoughts of the past, both distant and recent, and live fully in the present.

- The Ego: It is one of the biggest hurdles to overcome to achieve lasting peace. The ego is the sense of "I-ness" or "my-ness" that manifests as selfishness and a feeling of separation from the world. Dissimulation, hypocrisy, exaggeration and secretiveness are traits of a dominant ego. A powerful ego clouds the intellect. Try to introspect and accept shortcomings. Be easy on yourself and have compassion when you discover personality aspects your ego would rather not see. Change will come with acceptance. With regular meditation and strong determination, you will be able to subdue ego and develop a powerful and selfless will.

As the practice deepens (experienced practitioners) you experience:

- Light: Different lights can appear in the mind during meditation. Bright white lights or a light of many colors, including yellow, red, blue, green and purple, can manifest. With time, they will remain for up to 30 minutes depending on the strength and degree of concentration. Try to keep a steady posture and breathe slowly, taking breaks if the intensity is too much. With constant practice, the phenomenon will grow familiar.

- Inner sounds: Anahata sounds are the mystic inner sounds heard during deep meditation. This is a sign of purification of the nadis (psychic nerve channels) due to sustained practice of prānāyāma. Anahata sounds are heard through the right ear and are loudest when both ears are held closed. To do this, sit cross-legged, blocking your ears with your thumbs, your eyes with your forefingers and your nostrils with your middle fingers. Pinch your mouth shut with your ring and little fingers. This is called Yani Mudra. Listen attentively to hear the mystic sounds, which are vibrations of prana in the heart.

- Visions of the astral plane: You may have visions of beings belonging to the astral plane. These beings are similar to those of the physical world but without a physical overcoat. They have subtle bodies with powers of materialization and dematerialization and can move about freely. They may appear to encourage or test you.

- Holy vision: Your ishta devata, the aspect of the Absolute to whom you are devoted, may appear to you in meditation practice. You will feel light, bliss, knowledge and divine love. You may have conversations with Him or Her. Once you attain cosmic consciousness, these conversations will stop. You will savor the language of silence, the language of the heart.

- Astral travel: You may experience a feeling of separation from your body during meditation practice. This will bring joy mixed with anxiety. You may experience a sensation of floating or rotating in an atmosphere filled with objects, beings and golden light. You will glide back into your physical body smoothly. Once you have experienced this, you will desire to return to the astral plane because your first experience might last only a few minutes. With patience, perseverance and firmness in practice, you will be able to leave your body at will and spend some hours in the astral plane. You will understand that you are not your body and that you have an existence outside the physical plane.

## Techniques of Relaxation/Meditation

There are many meditation techniques. Please experience them and find one that resonates to you and continue that tradition for the rest of your practice.

Bija mantra meditation: This was experienced and developed by Vishnu Divananda of Sivananda Vedanta Centers. Here is the sequence leading to the meditation.

1. Chant "Om" several times or even for a few minutes.

2. Draw attention to a long inhalation and exhalation and experience the subtleness of the expansion of the abdomen and chest.

3. Then, breathe normally until you barely notice the breath. Bring attention to the third eye (ajna chakra). A light may appear. Make sure not to judge; simply observe everything unfold in front of the third eye.

4. Repeat the mantra of the universe, "Om," or your personal mantra; synchronize the mantra with your breath. The mantra protects those who travel into the astral plane.

5. Repeat steps 2 to 4. If there is an intruding thought about anything in your life or in your imagination, then make a mental note and let it go, or count every thought that arrives. This normally stops the thought process.

6. Continue to dwell in this vast emptiness of space and meditative state for about 30 minutes or so.

7. Bring your attention back by chanting "Om" three times and chant the peace mantra for world peace, peace within and peace without.

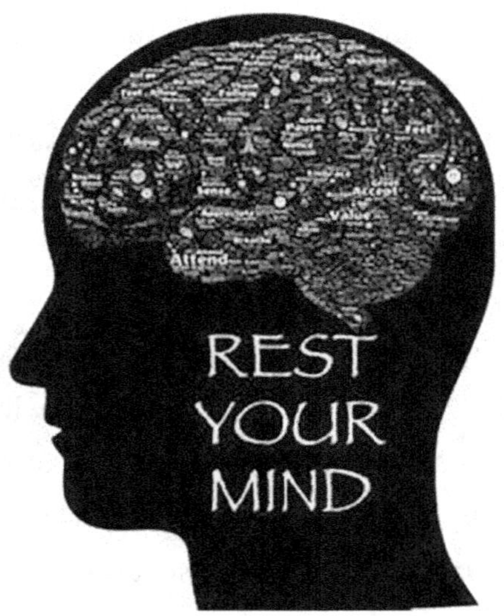


## Progressive Muscular Relaxation

Start focusing on breath and feel the rising and falling of your abdomen while inhaling and exhaling for a few breaths. Inhale and lift your right foot a couple inches off the floor and tense the entire right leg muscles. Exhale and release your muscles, letting go of all the tension. Inhale and lift your left leg and tense the muscles. Exhale and release. Inhale and tense your buttocks. Exhale and release. Inhale and push your lower back into the floor and tense your abdomen. Exhale and release. Inhale and lift your chest off the floor and push your shoulder blades together. Exhale and release. Inhale and lift both your arms off the floor. Tense the arms, make fists, bring your shoulders to your ears and push your shoulders away from ears. Exhale and release. Inhale and bring all your face muscles into your nose, then open your face and mouth, stick your tongue out and look up and back. Exhale and release. Inhale and push your neck into the floor. Exhale and release. Inhale, then exhale and turn your head to the right and hold the position for another breath. Inhale and bring your head to the center. Exhale and turn your head to the left and hold the position for another breath. Inhale and bring your head back. Exhale and bring your chin slightly towards your chest, and stay this position and relax for a few minutes.

## Autosuggestion

Every action is the result of a thought originating in the mind consciously and unconsciously. Thoughts take form in action and the body reacts to it. Autosuggestion is a relaxation technique where you suggest that your muscles and internal organs relax. Start by focusing on your breath and feel the abdomen rise and fall for a few breaths. Bring your awareness to your lower legs and start relaxing your toes, ankles, feet, calves, shins, knees, thighs, buttocks, hips and pelvis. The lower legs are relaxed. Bring your awareness to your upper body and start relaxing your abdomen, chest, lower back, mid and upper back, shoulders, upper arms, elbows, forearms, wrists, palms and fingers. The upper body is relaxed. Bring your awareness to the head region and start relaxing your chin, cheeks, mouth, lips, tongue, nose, eyes, eyebrows, forehead, ears and scalp. The head region is relaxed. Now bring your awareness to your internal organs and start relaxing your heart, lungs, liver and intestines. Your internal organs are relaxed. Stay in this relaxed state for a few minutes.

## Mental Relaxation

The constant tension on the mind due to unnecessary worries and anxieties takes away more energy than physical tension. When experiencing mental tension, breathe slowly and rhythmically for a few minutes and concentrate on breathing. Slowly, the mind will become calm and you can feel a kind of floating sensation, as if one were as light as a feather, then one feels peace and joy.

## Out-of-Body Relaxation

Some texts refer to out-of-body-relaxation as spiritual relaxation. As long as one identifies oneself with the body and mind there are no worries, sorrows, anxieties, fear and anger, which in turn bring tension. Yoga philosophy says that unless you withdraw from bodily cravings and sensations and separate yourself from ego consciousness, you cannot obtain complete relaxation. Therefore, through physical and mental relaxation, one may be led to spiritual relaxation: relaxation without thoughts, dramas, sensations, forms, names, times and symbols. You then experience out-of-body-relaxation.

## Vipasana Meditation

Vipasana meditation was experienced and developed by a Buddhist monk from Myanmar. It gained global popularity when a regimen of 10 days of silent meditation in a residential facility was introduced. It focuses on breath from one area of the body at a time, moving from the top of the head to the bottom of the feet and then reverses in direction. One continues the cycle for as many times as needed.

## Meditation in Nature

When you travel to or are lucky enough to live close to nature, learn to meditate on all senses of the environment, for example, the sounds of birds, waterfalls, waves, even animals and people, the smell of flowers, forests and rain. Let your mind and body go, without judging, and simply witness the beauty around you and in you. Finally, delve into the vast emptiness of the universe.

## Meditation in Five Essential Elements

Focus on the elements of the universe: earth, water, fire, air and ether, inside and outside the body to fully experience the elements in detail. Focus without letting thoughts interrupt your concentration. Then, eventually you will enter the meditative stage.

## Meditation on Perceptional State

Simply delve into a perceptual state of four power animals or your personal power animal(s), feel the energy of the archetypes and become the essence of the serpent, jaguar, hummingbird and eagle or condor. Let the archetype take you anywhere and anyplace, without judgment and fear, simply experience the beauty of another dimension of existence.